Injury Control

To Sara,
With best wishes
for a splendid
adventure in
Africa!
Larry Berger
5/14/96

Injury Control
A Global View

LAWRENCE R. BERGER
DINESH MOHAN

Foreword by

Dr C. J. ROMER
Chief, Injury Prevention Programme, WHO

DELHI
OXFORD UNIVERSITY PRESS
BOMBAY   CALCUTTA   MADRAS
1996

Oxford University Press, Walton Street, Oxford OX2 6DP

Oxford New York
Athens Auckland Bangkok Bombay
Calcutta Cape Town Dar es Salaam Delhi
Florence Hong Kong Istanbul Karachi
Kuala Lumpur Madras Madrid Melbourne
Mexico City Nairobi Paris Singapore
Taipei Tokyo Toronto
and associates in
Berlin Ibadan

ISBN 0 19 563680 5

Typeset by Rastrixi, New Delhi 110070
Printed in India at Pauls Press, New Delhi 110020
and published by Neil O'Brien, Oxford University Press
YMCA Library Building, Jai Singh Road, New Delhi 110001

Foreword

This book, which was initiated and supported by the WHO Injury Prevention Programme provides an overview of the current status and trends of injuries in countries throughout the world. It also discusses the value and limitations of injury data, the scientific basis of injury research and control, and the role of health professionals in addressing injuries as a public health problem. The book is primarily intended for teachers and students in medicine and public health, practicing physicians and other health care providers, and individuals who are serving as (or soon will become!) co-ordinators of community injury control programmes.

During the past few years, research on injuries has increased dramatically. Previously, many health professionals did not consider injury prevention a priority. Except for surgeons, physicians have been more concerned with diseases than injuries (a very questionable distinction, discussed in Chapter 6). Furthermore, much of injury prevention involves community approaches (passing laws, conducting educational campaigns) or engineering solutions that are outside the traditional medical arena. Insufficient funding, few scientists and teachers trained in injury control, involvement with previously-identified major medical problems (such as malnutrition, vaccine-preventable diseases, and AIDS), the belief that most injuries are random events or 'acts of God' that are not preventable, and a lingering perception that injury control is not a 'legitimate' medical or public health discipline, have also contributed to the neglect of injuries.

This book offers an alternative view: injuries are a profoundly important medical and public health problem; they are preventable, often by currently available technologies and strategies; and health professionals have a very important role to play in their prevention. The book's major emphasis is on unintentional injuries. Intentional injuries (suicide, homicide, rape, child abuse, spouse violence); politically sponsored injuries (civil strife, torture, and warfare); and injuries from natural disasters receive only limited discussion. This decision is based on expediency, our desire to limit the length of the text. The principles of injury analysis and control apply to all injuries.

The basic principles of analysis and approaches to injury prevention are universal. The influence of environmental and cultural factors, however, is best seen in a cross-national context. There is much to be learnt from examining the injury problems, successes, and mistakes of different countries. The highly industrialized countries (HICs) have documented the need to set limits on toxic exposures (such as the amount of lead in paints and gasoline), the value of motor vehicle safety standards, the importance of injuries in occupational health, and the effectiveness of automatic protection in reducing injuries, rather than an exclusive reliance on educational approaches. The injury profiles of the less-industrialized countries (LICs) emphasize the importance of pedestrian injuries, occupational injuries involving children (especially in the agricultural setting), and the acute and chronic hazards of pesticides. Injury research in LICs has often highlighted the value of low-cost, yet very effective, injury reduction strategies.

Another reason for examining injuries in both HICs and LICs is that injury problems have become multinational in scope. Pesticides used by South American farmers appear in foods on dinner tables in Europe and North America; automobiles made in Japan, Korea, and the USA traverse the roads of Thailand and Argentina; toxic chemical release from a factory owned by a foreign based company; airborne radiation from Chernobyl (former USSR) affected dairy farms in Scandinavia. In many ways, it is impossible to avoid a global perspective on injury control.

This book is not intended to be the definitive reference on injuries. It is a learning instrument, addressing basic concepts that are illustrated through numerous examples, diagrams, and photographs. Because our focus is on *prevention*, there is little said about the treatment and rehabilitation of injury victims. Even when clinical issues, such as the pathophysiology of injuries, are discussed, it is in the context of how such knowledge contributes to designing effective prevention strategies. There already exist many excellent references on critical care medicine. Hopefully, this book will fulfill the desire of health professionals for a concise review of topics related to injury prevention and control in an international context. Other key references, listed in Appendix A, discuss in more depth the topics which can only be briefly summarized in this work. Ideas and curricula for incorporating injury control topics into a variety of educational settings are increasingly available.[1-4]

We hope this book will stimulate enthusiastic discussions, further reading, and additional research in injury control. We have-chosen not to divide chapters by injury problems (falls, drownings, poisonings, occupational injuries, intentional injuries, etc.). Instead, the most important topics appear in different chapters as illustrations of broader principles of injury control (interpreting data, using comparison groups, automatic protection, and so on). Chapter One offers an overview of injury problems in different countries, emphasizing how the patterns of injury differ between the rich and poor nations. Obtaining and interpreting data about injuries is the subject of Chapter Two; Chapter Three reviews methodologic issues in conducting original epidemiologic research on injuries, including programme evaluation. The contribution of biomechanics, anatomy, and physiology to injury prevention are illustrated in Chapter Four. Chapter Five contains important topics relating to developmental, behavioural and social aspects of injury. Approaches to injury prevention, especially the role of the health sector are the subject of the last two chapters. The 'Afterword' offers thoughts on the future of injury control as a field for research and action.

CLAUDE J. ROMER, M.D.,
Chief, Injury Prevention Programme
World Health Organization

REFERENCES

1. Berger, L. R. 1991. Education and training in injury control. In: Manciaux, M., Romer, C. J. (eds), *Accidents in Childhood and Adolescence: The Role of Research*, WHO, Geneva, Chapter 15, pp. 173–88.
2. Holden, J. A., Christoffel, T. A course for health professionals on motor vehicle trauma. For information, contact Janet A. Holden, Ph.D, University of Illinois, School of Public Health, Box 6998, Chicago, IL 60680.
3. EPIC, 1991. *Educating Professionals in Injury Control*. Education Development Center, Inc. (EDC) and the Johns Hopkins Injury Prevention Center. For information, contact EDC, 55 Chapel Street, Newton, MA 01260 USA.
4. EDC, 1991. *Preventing Injuries* and *Violence Prevention*; Teenage Health Teaching Modules.

Acknowledgements

Dr Claude Romer, Director of the Global Injury Prevention Programme of the World Health Organization (WHO), originated the idea for this book, brought together its contributors, and made possible the collection of data from many countries and agencies. We received valuable material from Professor A. Got, Ambroise Pare Hospital, Paris; Dr Leif Svanstrom, Karolinska Institute, Stockholm; Richard J. Smith, Injury Control Division, Indian Health Service (USA), Rockville, Maryland; and Thavisak Svetsreni, Mahidol University, Bangkok.

Many other people provided ideas and information: Elias Anzola-Perez and Shrikant Bangdiwala (PAHO), Jose Jordan (Ministry of Public Health, Havana), Imrana Qadeer (Jawaharlal Nehru University, New Delhi), Murray Mackay (University of Birmingham, England), Gordon Trinca (Royal Australasian College of Surgeons, Melbourne), Dorothy Clemmer (Tulane University), Stewart Brown, Jerry Hershovitz, Mark Rosenberg, and Richard Waxweiler (CDC, Atlanta), Susan Baker, Gordon Smith, Stephen Teret and Modena Wilson (John Hopkins University), W. H. J. Rogmans (Netherlands Consumer Safety Institute), Maurice Backett (Lidstones, England), Vichit Punyahotra (Mahidol University, Bangkok), Janet Holden (University of Illinois, School of Public Health), Sylvia Micik (San Diego, California), Frederick Rivara (University of Washington, Seattle), Narayan Thapa (Kanti Children's Hospital, Kathmandu), Joseph Greensher (Roslyn, New York), Takeshi Hirayama (Tokyo Women's Medical College), and Garen Wintemute (Sacramento, California).

Jonathan A. Meyers of JAM Photography in Albuquerque expertly transformed Dr Berger's colour slides and prints into publishable black and white photographs. Illustrations were created by Jane Fleming, Sarah Langwell, Peggy McAfee, and Michael Norviel of the Medical Illustrations Department of the University of New Mexico. The faculty and staff of the Centre for Biomedical Engineering at the Indian Institute of Technology provided research support throughout the preparation of the manuscript. Mahesh K. Gaur was instrumental in maintaining all the computer files. Sarah Morley and Mary Strawn of the Lovelace Medical Library provided skilled bibliographic support. The authors are also grateful to many individuals and publishers for permission to reproduce text, tables, and illustrations.

It is not possible to thank everyone who shared valuable insights and information during the preparation of the manuscript. There is truly a global community of physicians, scientists, and other public servants whose devotion to public health transcends personal recognition and international borders. This book is dedicated to that community.

Contents

1

Overview

SCOPE OF THE INJURY PROBLEM

Each year, at least three and a half million people die from injuries around the world, more than two million in low-income countries (LICs).[1] Globally, about half of all deaths in the age group 10–24 years are due to injuries, intentional and unintentional.[2] For all ages, injuries rank fifth among the leading causes of death in the world and account for 10–30 per cent of all hospital admissions.[3, 4] An estimated 78 million persons are disabled each year because of injuries.[5]

Reports from various nations confirm that injuries are a major health problem throughout the world.

Thailand

Since 1969, injuries have been the leading cause of death in Thailand. The death rate has more than doubled between 1975 and 1981 (from 16 deaths per 100,000 population to 33). In 1983, nearly two million injured people were treated in hospitals with 31,000 deaths. Thirty per cent of hospital beds outside Bangkok are occupied by patients with injury. The economic burden of injuries is staggering—40,000 million Baht (US $1.5 billion) in direct costs alone in 1987.[6]

United States of America

From ages 1 to 44 years in the United States, deaths due to injury out number all other causes. For all ages, injuries are the third leading cause of death, with 150,000 injury fatalities each year.[7] The economic cost to the nation from unintentional injuries is an estimated $400 billion.[8]

China

China has an age-adjusted death rate from injuries (69 per 100,000 population in 1986) that exceeds that of the United States (61 per 100,000). The US has higher death rates from motor vehicle crashes, fires, and homicide. China has greater mortality from drowning, poisoning, falls, and suicide.[9]

India

Estimates of the number of annual deaths from injuries in India range from 130,000 to 650,000. About 15 per cent of all hospital beds are occupied by injury victims.[10] Over 10,000 deaths and one million disabling injuries annually are attributed to burns in India. In 1992 the Government of India reported more than 57,000 deaths from traffic injuries in the country.[11]

New Zealand

New Zealand had 58,457 hospital admissions and 1,250 deaths from unintentional injuries in 1983. Among persons aged 1–34 years, these injuries were the leading cause of death. A quarter of all fatal injuries were intentional.[12]

Middle East and Africa

In the Middle East and Africa during the mid-1980's, rising numbers of motor vehicles were taking an increasing toll. Traffic deaths per 100,000 population ranged from 2.5 in Ethiopia and 13.4 in Kenya, to 27.1 in Kuwait and 30.5 in South Africa (compared to 10.0 in Sweden).[13]

Latin America

By the early 1980's, injuries were the leading cause of death in the age group of 1–4 years in Argentina, Costa Rica, Cuba, Chile, Puerto Rico and Uruguay. For children ages 5–14 years, injuries were the leading cause of death in an additional 12 Latin American nations.[14] Among males between 20–24 years, injuries accounted for 71 per cent of all deaths in Cuba, 68 per cent in Venezuela, and 52 per cent in Costa Rica.[15]

While motor-vehicle related injuries (involving occupants, pedestrians, motorcyclists, and bicyclists) remain a leading cause of injury deaths, violence related injuries (homicides, assaults, rapes, child abuse) are increasing in importance.[16-19] The United States has a homicide rate ten times the rate of other Western nations, with about 300,000 homicide deaths annually. In Peru, wife abuse accounts for 75 per cent of police reports of assault. A study from Bangkok reported that 50 per cent of wives say they are 'regularly beaten' by their husbands.[1]

HICs AND LICs

United Nations publications often bisect the world into the 'less developed' and 'more developed' regions on the basis of demographic and other socio-economic indicators:

> The less developed regions include all regions of Africa, Asia (excluding Japan), Latin America and Oceania (excluding Australia and New Zealand). The more developed regions include all regions of Europe, The Union of Soviet Socialist Republics, Northern America, and the regions just cited as being outside the less developed category.[20]

The terms 'high-income countries' (HICs) and 'low-income countries' (LICs) are used throughout this book in place of 'developed' and 'developing' countries. 'Development' has connotations of social hierarchy that we prefer to avoid. High or low income emphasizes the powerful influence of a country's economic status on its patterns of injuries. Even a crude indicator like the gross national product (GNP) per capita can distinguish countries with vastly different social and economic circumstances. Arbitrarily dividing countries by whether their annual GNP per capita is greater or less than $3,000 results in the geographic picture seen in (Figure 1.1).[21, 22] This corresponds closely to the 'less developed/more developed' UN regions.

Assigning countries to broad categories obviously ignores the vast differences among nations in geography, occupations, cultural traits, political structures, and all the other characteristics that make each country unique. There is value to the approach, however, because countries of similar economic status share so many social and demographic characteristics. This is illustrated in (Table 1.1) comparing Kenya (a low-income country or 'LIC'), the Republic of Korea (a 'NIC'

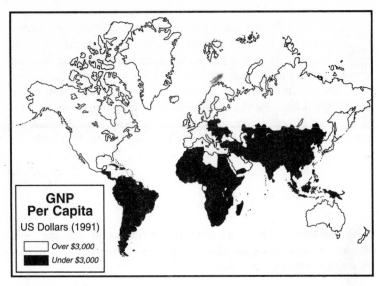

GNP Per Capita
US Dollars (1991)

☐ Over $3,000
■ Under $3,000

Figure 1.1: A North–South division is apparent in the economic status of nations. Based on data from the *World Development Report 1993: Investing in Health.* Published by Oxford University Press, New York for The World Bank, 1993.

Table 1.1
LICs, NICs and HICs (1991)

	Republic of Kenya	Republic of Korea (South)	Sweden
Population in millions	25	43	9
Per cent under 15 years old	49	25	18
GDP in billions of $ (US)	7.1	283	206
GNP per capita	$340	$6,330	$25,110
Per cent urban	24	73	84
Reported literacy rate	69	96	99
Population per physician	10,130	1,370	370
Infant mortality/1,000 births	67	16	6
Life expectancy at birth (yr)	59	70	78

Source: *World Development Report 1993: Investing in Health,* New York, Oxford University Press, 1993.

or newly-industrialized country), and Sweden (a high income country or 'HIC').[22] Levels of income, literacy rates, health indices, transport and communication infrastructures—are all interrelated and have a tremendous influence on the nature and extent of injuries in a country.

CIRCUMSTANCES OF INJURIES

The major types of injuries namely motor vehicle trauma, falls, drownings, poisonings, intentional violence are the same in almost all countries. However, the nature and extent of injuries will obviously vary

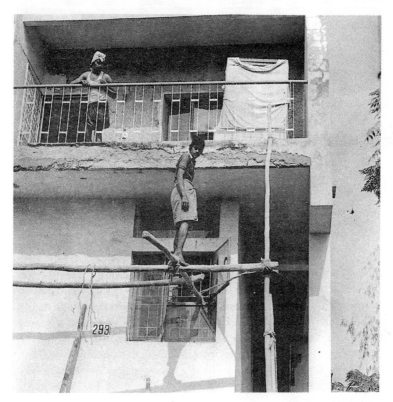

Photo 1.1: Falls are major problems in LICs. In the cities, many falls occur during house construction and repair. In rural areas, falls from trees are also common.

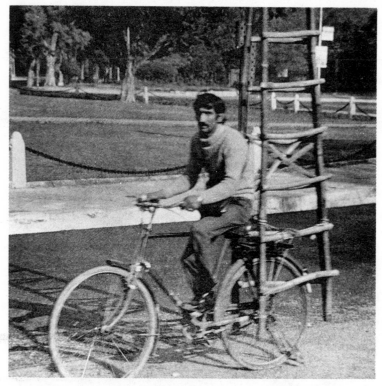

Photo 1.2: In HICs, bicycles are usually recreational vehicles.
In LICs, they are a basic means of transportation for people and goods.

according to geographic, cultural, urban/rural and other differences (Photos 1.1 and 1.2). Understanding these differences can greatly influence the choice of countermeasures. For example, a higher proportion of motor vehicle injuries involve motorcyclists and pedestrians in LICs. Mandatory seat belt laws and child safety device laws will, therefore, not have as great an impact in LICs as in HICs, where motor vehicle occupant deaths are more common. Burns in LICs are commonly caused by kerosene lamps and stoves, boiling water, and open fires. Lowering hot water heater temperatures, a recommendation for industrialized countries, makes little sense for households without electricity.

Examples of the most common injuries experienced in HICs and LICs and illustrations of groups at particularly high risk are summarized in (Table 1.2). Strategies to address these injuries are discussed in Chapter Six.

Table 1.2
Major Causes of Severe Injuries in HICs and LICs

LICs	HICs
Motor Vehicles	
Vulnerable road users (pedestrians, bicyclists, etc.) struck by motor vehicles.	Occupants of private automobiles involved in single and multiple-vehicle crashes.
Motorcycle crashes.	Motorcycle crashes.
People falling off and crashes of public transport vehicles (buses and trains).	Pedestrians (especially children and elderly) struck by cars.
Drivers of trucks killed in crashes.	Farm tractor rollovers.
Labourers falling from open truck beds.	Young people falling from recreational 'all-terrain' vehicles.
Fires and Burns	
Fires in slum and squatter housing.	House fires in private dwellings, especially in slum housing and mobile homes.
Scalds from boiling water.	Scalds from hot tap water, cooking gas and boiling water.
Explosion of pressurized stoves.	
Ignition of clothing by open cooking fires, kerosene lamps and pressurized stoves.	Ignition of clothing by cigarettes, outdoor fires, portable heaters.
Children falling into open cooking fires.	Occupational burns from molten metals, gasoline powered appliances/vehicles.
Drownings	
Children falling into open wells.	Children falling into home swimming pools.
Floods.	Leisure boat incidents.
Public transport on waterways.	Intoxicated persons near any body of water.

LICs	HICs
Bathing and drinking at lakes, ponds and rivers.	–

Falls

LICs	HICs
Workers from high trees: e.g., palm and coconut trees.	Children from apartment windows.
–	Children, elderly falling down stairs.
Children from rooftops, low trees, (e.g., fruit trees) and farm animals.	'Baby walker' devices.
Home construction and repair.	Elderly slipping on ice.
–	Construction workers.

Poisonings

LICs	HICs
Kerosene, gasoline and pesticides stored in household containers.	Household chemicals (e.g., drain cleaners).
Pesticide spraying by families.	Carbon monoxide from cars, home heaters.
Snake and insect bites.	Medications.
Environmental lead.	Environmental lead.
Plants (e.g., cassava).	Overdoses of alcohol and illegal drugs (heroin, cocaine).

Intentional Injuries

LICs	HICs
Suicides from ingesting liquid pesticides.	Suicides involving firearms or ingestion of medications.
Assaults and homicides.	Firearm related assaults/homicides.
Political and ethnic conflicts.	Military actions.
Domestic violence (e.g., dowry-burnings).	Child abuse, rape, domestic violence.

Agricultural Injuries

LICs	HICs
Pesticide exposures.	Pesticide exposures.
Chaff cutter and grain thresher amputations.	Farm tractor rollovers.
Drive-belt (patta belt) entrapment.	Farm machinery injuries.
Machette injuries.	–

LICs	HICs
Snake and animal bites; insect stings.	–

Non-Farm Occupational Injuries

LICs	HICs
Injuries from unprotected machinery.	Motor vehicle crashes.
Poisonings and burns from manufacture of chemicals.	Musculoskeletal disorders from cumulative trauma.
Falls.	Falls.
High-risk industries include mining, construction, small-scale manufacturing, ('unorganised sector', including child labour).	High-risk industries include coal mining, construction, lumber and sawmills, meat products, shipbuilding and repair, trucking.

INJURIES COMPARED TO OTHER CAUSES OF DEATH

In HICs, the greatest number of deaths occur among the elderly (Figure 1.2).[23] Improved economic conditions and advances in medical care have meant that many more people are living beyond 65

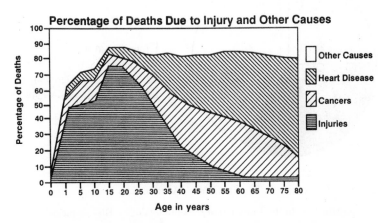

Figure 1.2: Mortality data from South Australia shows the importance of injuries relative to other major causes of death at different ages. Figure courtesy: Chris Baker, South Australia Department of Health.

years of age. Coupled with declining birth rates, these trends mean that the elderly constitute a larger proportion of the overall population in these countries.[24] Injuries, however, take their greatest toll in deaths among older children and young adults. The median age at death in the US is 27 years for motor vehicles, 32 years for homicide, 68 years for cancers, and 76 years for cardiovascular disease.[25] Therefore, on a total-population basis, injuries often follow heart disease, cancer, and stroke as a cause of death in HICs. When only 'premature' deaths are considered ('premature' being defined as deaths before the usual retirement age or before the age of average life expectancy), injuries lead all other causes.[26, 27] In New Zealand, for example:

> Life expectancy is approximately 70 years. Deaths prior to age 70 are sometimes referred to as premature, and the number of years of life that would have remained are considered years of life lost prematurely or 'potential years of life lost' (PYLL). The method of calculating PYLL involves summing for all age groups between 1 and 70 years the number of deaths in a specific age group multiplied by the remaining

Percentage of years of potential life lost to injury, cancer, heart disease, and other diseases before age 65*

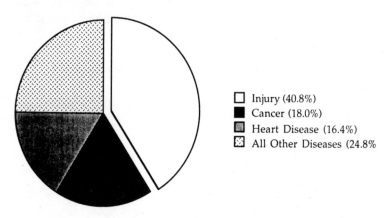

☐ Injury (40.8%)
■ Cancer (18.0%)
▨ Heart Disease (16.4%)
▧ All Other Diseases (24.8%)

* Source: Centers for Disease Control, Atlanta, GA.

Figure 1.3: In the United States, as in most other HICs, injuries make up the largest proportion of years of potential life lost (YPLL). From *Injury in America*, National Academy Press, Washington, D.C., 1985, p. 5. No copyright.

years of life up to age 70. Just over a quarter of all potential years of life lost are attributable to unintentional injuries.[12]

Results from a similar calculation of 'Years of Potential Life Lost' (YPLL) for the United States are displayed in (Figure 1.3).[7] For India, injuries rank second after infectious diseases when a YPLL calculation is done for all deaths of people more than four years of age.[10]

The demographic distribution of deaths in LICs is dramatically different from HICs. Infants and young children are the largest age group in terms of overall number of deaths. Nearly 40 per cent of all annual deaths in LICs are children under age 5 compared to 3 per cent in HICs. Of the 15 million children under age 5 who died annually in the years 1980–5, 98 per cent were in LICs, primarily in South Asia and Africa.[20] These deaths are the result of malnutrition, diarrhoeal and respiratory diseases, and other infections. Even in LICs, however, injuries need to be a public health priority because:

1. They are the leading cause of death and morbidity in the middle of the age spectrum (from age 4 or 5 years to 35 years and older in many LICs);
2. The incidence of specific injuries such as motor vehicle and occupational injuries is much higher in some LICs than in HICs; and,
3. Injuries will assume an ever higher proportion of total deaths in LICs in the future. Economic development, safe water supplies, and vaccination programmes reduce deaths from diarroheal diseases, viral diseases (measles, rubella, polio), acute respiratory infections, and nutritional deficiencies. Even with no change in incidence rates, injuries emerge as a leading cause of death (Figure 1.4).[7]

The decline of competing illnesses, however, is not the only reason that injuries have surfaced as an important cause of mortality and morbidity. Other major factors leading to increased injuries are urbanization, industrialization, and motorization. In the highly-industrialized countries, these developments occurred over more than half a century. In many LICs, the same drastic changes occur in less than a decade, without accompanying improvements in general economic conditions or national infrastructures (e.g., communications, roads, and medical services).

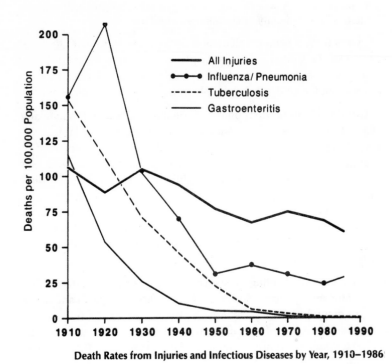

Death Rates from Injuries and Infectious Diseases by Year, 1910–1986

Figure 1.4: Dramatic declines in death rates from infectious diseases in the United States were not accompanied by a similarly sharp fall in injury death rates. From Baker, S. P., O'Neill, B., Ginsburg, M. J., Li, G., *The Injury Fact Book*, Oxford University Press, New York, 1992, p. 11. Copyright 1992 by Oxford University Press, Inc.

URBANIZATION

It is well known that many LICs are experiencing high rates of population growth. Between 1960 and 1980, the population of the world increased by 46 per cent, from 3 billion to nearly 4.5 billion. By the year 2000, the world's population is projected to be over six billion people, with 4.85 billion (80 per cent) living in LICs. Less well-known is the extraordinary rapid urbanization that is occurring (Figure 1.5).[28] The population of cities has grown more than twice as fast as the total

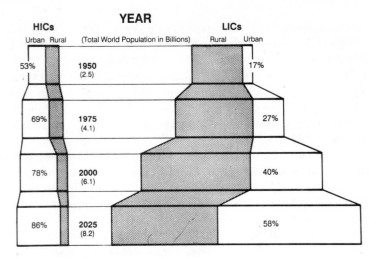

Figure 1.5: Actual and projected changes in population growth and urban/rural distribution in HICs and LICs. The widths of the figures are proportional to the actual number of people. In the year 2025, the projected world population will be 8.2 billion, with 6.8 billion people living in LICs. 86% of people in HICs and 58% in LICs will be living in urban areas. From, The World's Urban Explosion, *The Courier*, UNESCO, March, 1985, pp. 24–9.

Table 1.3
Ten Largest Urban Centres in the World (1990)

		Population (millions)
1.	Mexico City	20.2
2.	Tokyo/Yokohama	18.1
3.	Sao Paulo	17.4
4.	Greater New York	16.2
5.	Shanghai	13.4
6.	Los Angeles	11.9
7.	Calcutta	11.8
8.	Greater Buenos Aires	11.5
9.	Bombay	11.2
10.	Seoul	11.0

Source: *World Development Report 1993: Investing in Health*, New York, Oxford University Press, 1993.

world population during the past twenty years.[29] From 1900 to 1975, the number of cities with over five million inhabitants increased by a factor of twenty the total population of the twenty-five largest cities more than quadrupled. Major cities are adding hundreds of thousands of people to their populations each year—350,000 in Cairo, 300,000 in Bangkok and 750,000 in Mexico City.[28] Each of the ten largest urban agglomerations in the world contains over 10 million people (Table 1.3).[22]

Rural/urban migration has been a major factor. However, more than half the urban increase is due to natural birth rates. Many cities are already unable to provide basic medical care, social services, employment, water, sewage disposal, housing and mass transit for vast numbers of residents. Serious overcrowding and inadequate infrastructure contributes to traffic injuries, alcohol and drug addiction, mental illness, and violence. The impact is particularly severe for children. Violent deaths are common, for example, among the street children (gamines) of Bogota and other cities.[30]

Of the 1.3 billion children in developing countries, almost half will spend their entire lives in temporary slum shelters that are often nothing more than discarded packing crates and cardboard boxes. Increasing numbers are being abandoned by impoverished and disenfranchised parents. In Brazil alone it is estimated that there are 11 million street children. Another 14 million who do have families are nevertheless growing up in conditions of extreme urban poverty.[31]

In many LICs, slum and squatter dwellers already represent 50–75 per cent of the urban population.[30] Squatters are "illegal" occupants of urban land. Slums are the oldest, most dilapidated housing in a city. Large squatter settlements, favelas, bidonvilles, hutments, bustees, villa miseries, house the majority of urban poor in many LICs. These settlements (Photo 1.3) are often located on railway embankments (New Delhi), swampy land (Bangkok), or precarious hillsides (Hong Kong)—putting their residents at great risk from floods, mudslides, and other natural disasters. The high population density of slums and settlements means that events like fires and toxic chemical releases can also have a devastating impact. Recent examples are the earthquake in Mexico City, the volcano and subsequent mudslides in Colombia, the nuclear power plant disaster at Chernobyl, USSR, and the release of toxic gases from a Union Carbide plant in Bhopal, India.

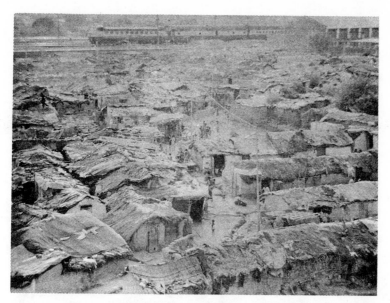

Photo 1.3: A squatter settlement in New Delhi.

INDUSTRIALIZATION

Industrialization is occurring in both rural and urban settings with a dramatic increase in the number and severity of injuries. Family-based, subsistence agriculture has given way to mechanization, rural electrification, and the widespread use of pesticides (Photo 1.4). Industrialization in the cities has meant the introduction of hazardous machinery, toxic chemicals, and high-rise construction.

Most of the workforce in LICs is involved in agriculture. Animal and human energy is being replaced by a large number of implements and machines powered by small engines or tractors. Engine-driven equipment operates at higher energies than human- or animal-powered equipment and, therefore, can inflict more severe injuries (Figure 1.6). To keep prices as low as possible, much of this equipment is sold without safety features. Most LICs have experienced a sharp increase in amputations, crushing of limbs, and electrocutions among their rural populations.

Agricultural chemicals, especially pesticides, have also caused havoc in many rural communities (see also Chapter 5). Many

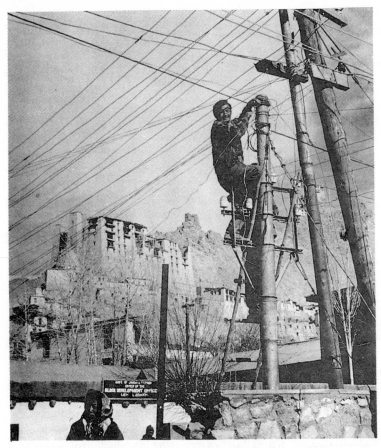

Photo 1.4: Electrification of rural areas brings with it electrical hazards for both workers and the general population.

governments in LICs have not been able to adequately control the manufacture or sale of highly toxic pesticides that are banned or whose use is severely restrictly in HICs. Many LICs have also been unable to promote the safe use of pesticides, since rural people are often powerless, may not know the long term effects of pesticides, and protective devices (masks, gloves, footwear, etc.) are too expensive for poor farmers. The widespread availability of the most toxic pesticides has also resulted in high rates of successful suicides. In Sri Lanka, suicide (primarily by ingestion of pesticides) is the

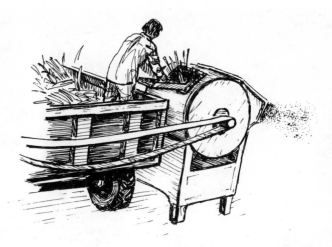

Figure 1.6: A motorized threshing machine. The power take-off belt appears in the foreground. If the farmer slips, his arm can enter the grain chute and become amputated.

leading cause of death among young people in the age group 15–24 years (see Exercise 4).

Many products, from bicycles to farm machinery, are made in small workshops or home based work units in LICs (Photo 1.5). This decentralization makes it very difficult to enforce safety standards and to monitor the quality and safety of products. Small workshop owners find it too costly to change equipment frequently; unsafe equipment, once purchased, remains in place for a long time. Equipment, such as printing presses or lathes, becomes more hazardous in LICs because of crowded workplaces, and inadequate lighting and ventilation. Improvements in health and safety are even more difficult to achieve in home-based industries, where workers have very little control over the production process. Beedies, inexpensive cigarettes made by wrapping tobacco in leaves, are made in Asia by women working at home. They are not organized as a workforce, so their piece-rate work for wholesalers is very demanding and very low-paying. They have to work long hours in uncomfortable postures, inhaling tobacco dust. Chemicals from the tobacco leaves damage the skin. Although the problems faced by beedi workers have been publicized for decades, there has been little improvement in their working conditions.

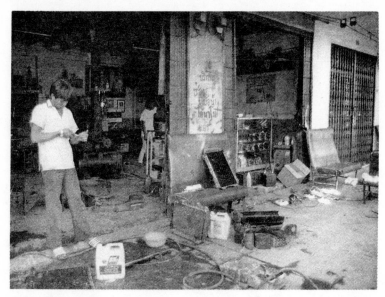

Photo 1.5: This radiator-repair shop in Bangkok is one of thousands of small businesses employing just a handful of workers. Enforcing labor laws in the 'unorganized sector' is extraordinarily difficult.

Large-scale industries in LICs also lack the safeguards that are routinely expected in HICs.[32, 33] The urgency to promote economic activity; the presence of a low-paid, poorly-educated, and non-unionized labour force; the scarcity of labour inspectors; and the pressure to keep costs low, all mean that workers' health and safety are often sacrificed. Machine maintenance is costly, so it is performed less frequently or not at all. At the same time, equipment is used for many more years in LICs than in HICs, increasing the chances for dangerous breakdowns. The large proportion of migrant workers and child labourers also increases injury rates because migrants are unable to exercise social or political influence over decision makers.

MOTORIZATION

Motorization refers to the influx of motor vehicles, including high-performance cars, trucks, and motorcycles, without concomitant

changes in roads, pedestrian patterns, or traffic enforcement capabilities. Although the bicycle continues to be the world's leading
vehicle for personal transportation (more than 100 million bicycles
were produced in 1992, 36 million in China alone),[34] the global increase in automobiles has been truly staggering (Figure 1.7).[35] Yet, as
these streams of motorcycles, buses, trucks, and cars appear, they
share the road with very old, slow moving vehicles including human-
and animal powered ones (Photo 1.6). The vast majority of road users,
pedestrians, riders or pullers of 'rickshaws' and carts, motorcyclists,
and bicyclists, are unprotected. In any collision with three or four-
wheeled vehicles, these road users sustain severe injuries. In many
LICs, motorcycles are the most popular form of family transportation
(Photo 1.7). Compared to automobiles, they are much cheaper to
purchase and maintain, and provide much better mileage per litre of

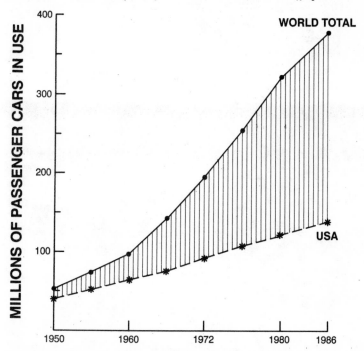

Figure 1.7: World production of motor vehicles has increased steadily
since 1950, with the United States assuming a much smaller share of the
total. Figure adapted from data in Table 6.1, in *State of the World 1989*,
p. 98, copyright Worldwatch Institute.

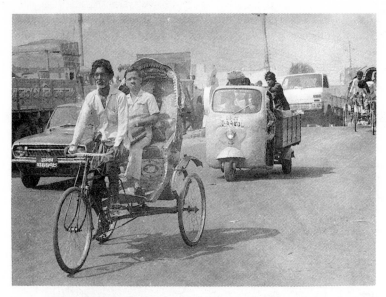

Photo 1.6: Bicycle rickshaws compete with various forms of motorized traffic on this street in Dhaka, Bangladesh.

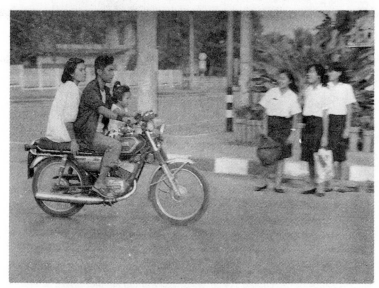

Photo 1.7: The motorcycle has become the family vehicle in many LICs. Mandatory helmet laws for drivers and passengers are still uncommon, however.

fuel. Yet motorcycle riders have the highest probability of dying in a crash—more than four times that of automobile or bus occupants in Delhi.[36]

Public transportation is vital in LICs, because most people are too poor to own personal vehicles. With increasing population growth and urbanization, public transportation systems are not able to keep up with the demand. Within cities, people often ride while hanging from open bus doors and on intercity routes, they will often sit on the roof of buses. Traumatic injuries in such situations are not uncommon. Burma has a particularly serious problem, in that passengers leave and enter at the *rear* of the bus (Photo 1.8). In a rear collision, passengers can suffer leg amputations or death. In Bangladesh, where many roads are interrupted by rivers and lakes, overloaded buses, sometimes with unsafe brakes, drive onto ferries with inadequate guardrails (Photo 1.9). Many people drown if the bus rolls into the water. Another type of hazard involving public transportation exists in Bangkok. Due to extreme congestion in the central streets, special lanes have been created where buses drive *opposite* to the

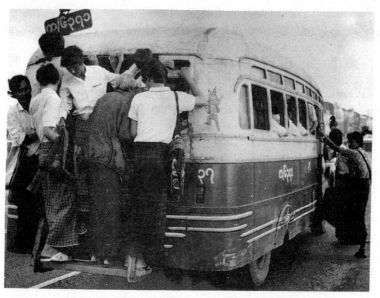

Photo 1.8: Doors at the rear of Rangoon buses mean that passengers riding outside are subject to amputations or worse in the event of rear-end collisions.

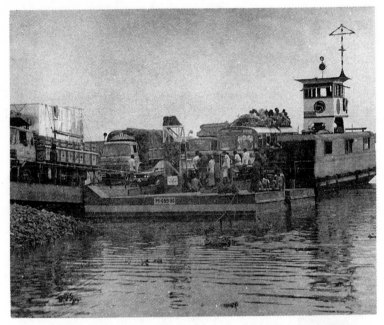

Photo 1.9: A ferry unloads at a dock in Bangladesh. A bus waits its turn to drive off with almost as many people on its roof as inside.

rest of the traffic flow (Photo 1.10). Woe to the pedestrian who forgets to look both ways before crossing a street in downtown Bangkok.

An additional problem for LICs are the new vehicles being manufactured in HICs with high acceleration rates. These very fast vehicles, especially high-powered motorcycles, are often driven at top speed on crowded city streets and narrow intercity roads. Few LICs have chosen to place engine-size restrictions on imported vehicles. Even when vehicles are manufactured by LICs for their domestic market, safety features are often lacking. The Maruti Gypsy, made in India, is patterned after Japan's Suzuki Samurai, a vehicle whose short wheel base and high centre of gravity are associated with deaths from roll-overs.[37] Most motorized vehicles in LICs have never been crash-tested or otherwise evaluated for safety before being mass produced (Photo 1.11). Some vehicles, especially in rural areas, are fabricated in small workshops and lack even the most basic safety features, such as headlights, quality brakes, or reliable steering mechanisms. Table 1.4 summarizes why LICs often have higher rates of motor vehicle injuries per vehicle than HICs.

Table 1.4
Some Factors Contributing to High Rates of Motor
Vehicle Injuries in LICs

High proportion of children and youth in the population.

Roads not paved and poorly maintained.

People and vehicles often not separated.

Roads used for vending, playing, and walking as well as driving vehicles.

Mix of vehicles with widely varying speeds.

Absence of standard safety features in vehicles (e.g., seat belts, quality brakes).

High proportion of motorcycles.

Vehicles poorly maintained.

Vehicle use extended beyond intended life of vehicle.

Few traffic police for licensing, inspection, enforcement of laws.

Poor or absent road illumination.

Absent land markings.

Lane markings applied to roads are subject to rapid deterioration because of heavy road use and climate (moisture, heat).

Deteriorated trucks commonly used in labour-intensive, low-investment industries to transport workers as well as supplies.

Unskilled drivers.

Pedestrians, especially children and recent migrants to the cities, unfamiliar with traffic behavior.

Walkers, bicyclists, and motorcyclists often carry burdens that interfere with vision and maneuverability.

Short tyre life because of driver behaviour and the tropical climate.

Rural police lack telephones or reliable electric power.

Motorcycles used for family transportation with up to five people per vehicle.

Inferior materials used for wheel bearings, brake pads, steering systems.

Overload of vehicles—public and private—with passengers.

Vegetation control and drainage cleaning are often not performed, resulting in flooded roads and warnings signs hidden by vegetation.

No shoulders next to roads.

Roadside hazards include drainage ditches and trees for shade.

Emergency medical systems often non-existent.

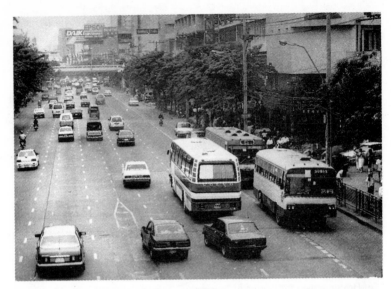

Photo 1.10: On this major Bangkok street, six lanes of traffic head in one direction, while one lane (intended for buses only) proceeds in the opposite direction adjacent to the sidewalk. Pedestrians who fail to look both ways before stepping into the street run a high risk of being run over by a bus.

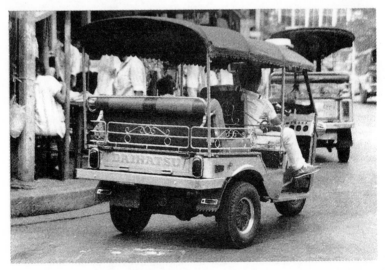

Photo 1.11: A propane-powered three-wheeled taxi (tuk-tuk) in Bangkok. The propane tank is directly beneath the rear passenger seat.

POVERTY AND INJURIES IN LICs

Poverty has a profound influence on all types of injuries. The great majority of people in LICs live in extreme poverty. More than half of the world's population lives in global regions where the per capita income is less than $500 a year.[21] Even when a country's per capita income is relatively high, the skewed nature of income distribution means that most people are still desperately poor. When families cannot afford transportation or medical care, minor injuries often become major ones. Without prompt treatment, a burn at the elbow can lead to contractures and a non-functioning limb. A foreign body in the eye can become infected and produce blindness. The child in Photo 1.12 had a fracture of his forearm that was not set; two years later, he was admitted to have his arm re-fractured in an attempt to improve the functional outcome. Emergency services and hospitals are in short supply in LICs; rehabilitation resources (prostheses, physical therapists, etc.) are virtually non-existent in many locations.

Poverty and its concomitants of illiteracy and powerlessness also influence injuries on a national scale. Safety devices and procedures required in industrialized countries, such as seat belts in cars, guards

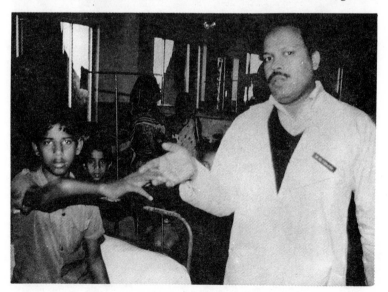

Photo 1.12: A young boy whose fractured arm was never set must have it re-broken two years later to improve function of the arm and hand.

around moving belts and rotors of factory machines, bans on extremely toxic pesticides, are often lacking in LICs (Photos 1.13 and 1.14). The high priority placed on economic development means that features or approaches that involve extra costs, either to the indigenous government or to investing companies, are often sacrificed. The public often remains unaware of the special risks associated with many new products, especially agricultural and household chemicals.

Injury control approaches that perform well in HICs can fail in LICs because of economic factors. For example, in Jakarta, Indonesia, bus passengers were being killed and injured when they fell from open doors. Buses with automatically-closing doors were introduced to prevent the falls. The automatic door mechanisms soon had to be

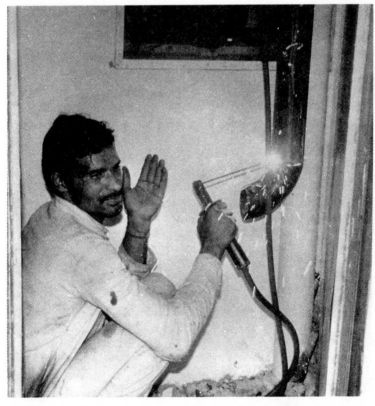

Photo 1.13: This welder in New Delhi has no protection fo his face, head, hands, or feet.

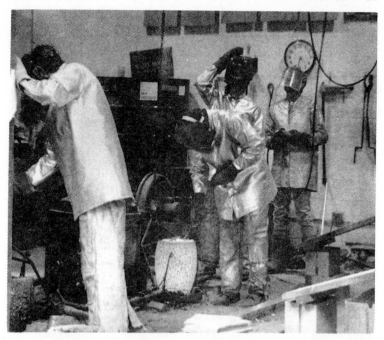

Photo 1.14: Unlike the welder in Photo 1.11, these workers wear heavy boots and gloves, asbestos suits, and massive helmets with visors for pouring molten bronze.

disconnected: the buses were so crowded, the doors usually could not close to allow the vehicles to move. However, similar measures are seen to work in overcrowded buses in China.

Nowhere is the influence of poverty more clear than for children, who comprise a much greater proportion of the population in LICs than in HICs (Table 1.5).[24] Cooking, heating, and illumination are provided by open fires or kerosene stoves and lamps that are on or close to the ground. Homes are often flimsy, flammable shelters that are susceptible to fires and natural disasters such as cyclones, floods, and earthquakes. Even the places where children play are dangerous such as: parental worksites littered with rubble, tools, pesticides, or construction material; busy roads; and even garbage dumps. One example of a household injury unique to poor families in Sri Lanka are the burns children suffer when they unintentionally shatter kerosene lamps made of discarded light bulbs (Photo 1.15). The fragile bulbs are used because they are inexpensive and require only one or two cents worth of kerosene to fill. A bottle lamp, slightly sturdier and equally inexpensive, requires three or four cents worth of kerosene. Two or three pennies are enough of a disincentive for many families to choose the more dangerous light bulbs. Another example concerns falls into wells in rural areas. Wooden covers would prevent many toddlers from drowning. However, the costs, in terms of purchasing wood and diverting wood from other uses (such as fuel), are prohibitive for rural families.

Table 1.5
World Population Distribution, 1990

Area	Total pop. (thousands)	Per cent under 15 yrs	Per cent over 64 yrs
World	5,292,200	32	6
Asia	3,112,700	33	5
Africa	642,100	45	3
Europe	498,400	20	13
Latin America	448,100	36	5
USSR	288,600	25	10
Northern America	275,900	21	12
Oceania	26,500	26	9

Source: UN Population Fund: State of the World Population 1992; UN Department of Economic and Social Development: Report on the World Social Situation, 1993.

Child labour is a phenomenon with enormous implications for injuries among children and youth. The employment of children is wide-spread practice in many LICs, where the child's labour is often the only source of a family's income. Children can be found working as domestic servants, farm labourers, street vendors, and shop assistants in most LICs.[38] Injuries associated with child labour include deaths and disability from falls; poisoning from pesticides and heavy metals (especially lead); silicosis from mines and quarries; and burns, eye trauma, and orthopaedic disabilities.[39] Although most countries have laws against child labour, they are often poorly enforced (see Chapter 5). Even when children are not working, the virtual absence of day-care facilities in LICs and the shortage of schools and teachers

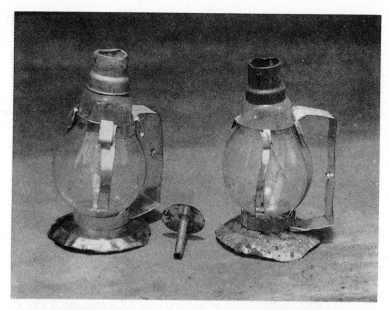

Photo 1.15: Discarded light bulbs are converted into kerosene lamps in rural Sri Lanka. The fragile glass is easily broken, especially by children playing on the floor, leading to burns and fires.

means that children often accompany their parents to construction sites, quarries, and farming locations, or are left at home with older siblings (Photo 1.16).

POVERTY AND INJURIES IN HICs

The economic discrepancy between rich countries and poor countries is enormous (Table 1.6).[22] Even within 'high-income' countries, however, there is usually a wide range of income from the poorest families to the most well-to-do. Socio-economic status plays a major role in determining the nature, frequency, and severity of injuries in HICs as well as in LICs. Yet socio-economic variables are often absent from injury statistics. The age, sex, and ethnic group are simpler variables to obtain than the income, occupation, or educational level of injury victims. The additional effort to record this data, however, is usually rewarded with important insights into factors related to

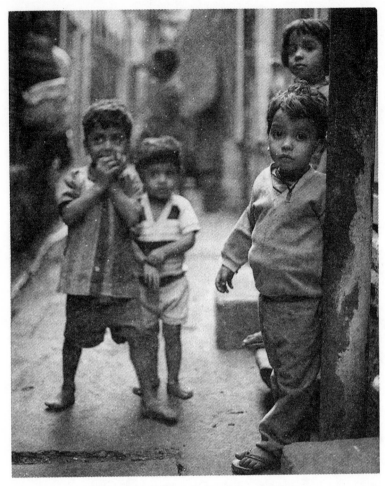

Photo 1.16: Children in the slums of LICs are
often unsupervised for large parts of the day.

injury causation. Studies in both the United States[40] and United Kingdom[41] show that overall injury death rates for children vary inversely
with the family's occupational status. Death rates from house fires,
which account for three-fourths of all deaths from fires and burns, are
more than twice as high in poverty areas.[42] Child pedestrian injuries
occur more often in poor neighbourhoods than in wealthier ones.[43]

Table 1.6
Countries with the Highest and Lowest
Reported GNP Per Capita (1991)

Countries	GNP per capita (US dollars)
Highest	
Switzerland	33,610
Japan	26,930
Sweden	25,110
Norway	24,220
Finland	23,980
Lowest	
Mozambique	80
Tanzania	100
Ethiopia	120
Uganda	170
Bhutan	180

Source: World Development Report 1993: Investing in Health. New York, Oxford University Press, 1993.

Reasons for children from low-income families in HICs having higher injury rates include:

1. Neighbourhood environment: higher density of both population and motor vehicle traffic, lack of protected play areas (such as parks and playgrounds), fire departments and/or rescue services often less well-equipped or staffed in poor communities,
2. Home environment: sub-standard housing with faulty heating and electrical systems, crowded rooms with inadequate escape routes, lead paint,
3. Social environment: less supervision from both parents working or single-parent household; care-takers with poor parenting skills; financial and social stresses increase risk of domestic violence,
4. Personal impact of poverty: hunger, illness, and inattentiveness; no shoes; no safety devices (such as car seats).

GLOBAL ACTION ON INJURIES

There is increasing recognition that injuries are a critical public health problem. When Thailand's National Safety Council (NSC) was formed, the Prime Minister agreed to become the president, lending vital political support for the NSC's efforts in motor vehicle, occupational, and domestic injury control. In the United States, the National Academy of Sciences issued a report describing injuries as 'the principal public health problem in America today'.[44] It called for 'an organized programme of effective action' to address injuries, including increased research, epidemiology, and training of health professionals in this field. As a result, the US National Highway Traffic Safety Administration (NHTSA) and the Centers for Disease Control (CDC) launched a co-ordinated effort for injury control in 1985, providing funding for five 'centers of excellence' at academic institutions and vastly expanding government research and training activities.

In India, new laws have been passed dealing with industrial safety (after the disastrous gas leak from the Union Carbide Plant in Bhopal), child labour, and motor vehicle safety. The country's Seventh Five-Year Plan included safety issues in the chapters on agriculture, employment, energy, industry, transport, and health and family welfare. Consumer protection groups have formed in most major Indian cities. India has a National Safety Council, Factory Safety Board, and National Institutes of Occupational Health and Toxicology Research. Both academic institutions and non-governmental organizations (such as the Indian Institute of Technology, Central Road Research Institute, and People's Science Institute) have targeted injuries as a health problem.

China has established large research institutes for worker safety and road safety. The Soviet Union also has many organizations studying injuries, including the Traumatology Research Institute. Indonesia has designated its Centre for Research on Non-Communicable Diseases as the lead agency for research on injuries. Brazil and Peru have groups involved in advocating for both urban and rural safety issues. Collaborating centres for research and action in the field of injury control have been established by the World Health Organization in countries around the world (Table 1.7). The Injury Prevention Programme of WHO also has co-sponsored world conferences on injury prevention and a 'Travelling Seminar on Safe Communities', where international participants visit model projects in both HICs and

LICs. Recently, an International Society of Child and Adolescent Injury Prevention (ISCAIP) has been organized 'to promote a significant reduction in the number and severity of injuries to children and adolescents through international collaboration.' The Society will provide a multi-disciplinary forum for research and advocacy.[45]

Table 1.7
WHO Collaborating Centres in Injury Control

Road Accident Research Unit
  National Health and Medical Research Council
  University of Adelaide
  Medicine Sociale et Preventive
  Faculte de Medicine
  Universite de Montreal

Centre Hospital-Universitaire Henri Mondor
  Service de Reeducation
  Paris

Centre de Medecine Geriatrique
  Universite Paul Sabatier
  Toulouse

Institut National de Recherche sur les Transports et leur Securite (INRETS)
  Arcueil Cedex

Centre for Biomedical Engineering
  Indian Institute of Technology
  New Delhi

Tokyo Women's Medical Research Institute
  Tokyo
Consumer Safety Institute
  Amsterdam

Department of Social Medicine
  Karolinska Institute
  Stockholm

Department of Plastic and Reconstructive Surgery
  Hacettepe University Medical School
  Ankara

Transport and Road Research Laboratory
Crowthorne

Center for Injury Control
Centers for Disease Control (CDC)
Atlanta

Southern California Injury Prevention Research Center
UCLA School of Public Health
Los Angeles

REFERENCES

1. World Health Organization Handle Life with Care, 1993. Prevent Violence and Negligence. World Health Day 1993, Information Kit, 7 April.
2. Friedman, H. L. 1985. The health of adolescents and youth: A global overview. *World Health Statistics Quarterly* **38**: 256–66.
3. Manciaux, M., Romer, C. J. 1986. Accidents in children, adolescents and young adults: A major public health problem. *World Health Statistics Quarterly* **39**: 227–31.
4. Global medium-term programme: Accident prevention, WHO, Geneva, APR/MTP/88.1, March 1988.
5. Stansfield, S. K., Smith, G. S., McGreevey, W. P. 1990. Injury and poisoning. In: Jamison, D. T., Mosley, W. H. (eds), *The World Bank Health Sector Priorities Review*, The World Bank, Washington, D.C., Chapter 24.
6. Accident and injury prevention at the primary health care level: Pattaya, Thailand, WHO, Geneva, 1987.
7. Baker, S. P., O'Neill, B., Ginsburg, M., Li, G. 1992. *The Injury Fact Book*. Second Edition, Oxford University Press, New York.
8. Accident Facts: 1993 Edition. National Safety Council, Itasca, IL, 1993.
9. Li, G., Baker, S. P. 1991. A comparison of injury death rates in China and the United States, 1986. *American Journal of Public Health* **81**: 605–9.
10. Mohan, D. 1984. Accidental death and disability in India: A stock-taking. Accident Analysis and Prevention **16**: 279–88.
11. Statistics of Road Accidents in India (1983–92). Ministry of Surface Transport, Government of India, New Delhi, 1993.
12. Langley, J., McLoughlin, E. A review of research on unintentional injury. Medical Research Council of New Zealand, Special Report Series No. 10, August 1987.
13. Trinca, G. W., Johnston, I. R., Campbell, B. J. et al. 1988. Reducing Traffic

Injury: A Global Challenge, Royal Australasian College of Surgeons, Melbourne.

14. A collaborative study of accidents in children and adolescents: Brazil, Chile, Cuba, and Venezuela, PAHO, Washington, D.C., August, 1987.

15. Manciaux, M., Taket, A. R. Accident mortality for young adults aged 20–4. Addendum to, Prevention of accidents in childhood and adolescence: Methodologies for research and programme monitoring and extent of the problem, WHO, Geneva, IRP/APR 216 m31K.4363E, October 1984.

16. Violence—a matter of health. 1993. *World Health* **1**: 1–31.

17. Rosenberg, M. L., Fenley, M. A. 1991. Violence in America, National Academy Press, Washington, D.C.

18. Bourbeau, R. 1993. Comparative analysis of violence death in the developed countries and in some developing countries, 1985–9. *World Health Statistics Quarterly* **46**: 1–5.

19. Mercy, J. A., Rosenberg, M. L., Powell, K. E. et al. 1993. Public health policy for preventing violence. *Health Affairs,* Winter **12**: 7–29.

20. Mortality of children under age five: World estimates and projections, 1950–2025, United Nations, New York, 1988.

21. United Nations Population Division: World population prospects, estimates and projections as assessed in 1982, United Nations, New York, 1985 (Population studies, No. 86).

22. World Development Report 1993: Investing in Health, Oxford University Press, New York, 1993.

23. South Australian Health Commission morbidity collection extracts, 1983.

24. UN Population Fund: State of the World Population 1992; UN Department of Economic and Social Development: Report on the World Social Situation, United Nations, New York, 1993.

25. Robertson, L. S. 1985. Trauma. In: Holland, W. W., Detels, Knox, G. (eds), *Oxford Textbook of Public Health:* Volume 4: Specific applications, Oxford University Press, Oxford, pp. 69–80.

26. Plaut, R., Roberts, E. 1989. Preventable mortality: Indicator or target? *World Health Statistics Quarterly* **42**: 4–15.

27. Rodriquez, L. A. G., daMotta, L. C. 1989. Years of Potential Life Lost: Application of an indicator for assessing premature mortality in Spain and Portugal. *World Health Statistics Quarterly* **42**: 50–4.

28. The world's urban explosion. The Courier, March 1985, UNESCO, Paris, pp. 24–9.

29. Yusof, K. 1984. Urban slum and squatter settlements: Variations in needs and strategies. In: Child Abuse and Urban Slum Environments. WHO/ISPCAN Pre-Congress Workshop Report, WHO, Geneva, pp. 4–19.

30. Manciaux, M. 1984. Urban slum and squatter settlements: Implications for child health. In: Child Abuse and Urban Slum Environments. WHO/ISPCAN Pre-Congress Workshop Report, WHO, Geneva, pp. 20–30.

31. Carballo, M. 1984. The emergence of urban slum and squatter settlements: A forum for child abuse. In: Child Abuse and Urban Slum Environments. WHO/ISPCAN Pre-Congress Workshop Report, WHO, Geneva, pp. 46–60.
32. Asogwa, S. E. 1987. Prevention of accidents and injuries in developing countries. *Ergonomics* **30**: 379–86.
33. Mohan, D. 1987. Injuries and the 'poor' worker. *Ergonomics* **30**: 373–7.
34. Ayres, E. 1993. Bicycle production resumes climb. In: Brown, L. F., Kane, H., Ayres, E. (eds), Vital Signs 1993, Worldwatch Institute, New York, pp. 86–7.
35. Renner, M. 1989. Rethinking transportation. In: Norton, W. W. (ed.), State of the World 1989, Worldwatch Institute, New York, pp. 97–112.
36. Mohan, D. 1993. Road traffic injuries in Delhi: Technology assessment, agenda for control. International Seminar on Road Safety, Srinagar, 1986, Indian Roads Congress, New Delhi.
37. Mohan, D. 1987. The Maruti syndrome: A disease of technological insecurity. *Business India* December 14–27, pp. 117–20.
38. Shah, P. M., Cantwell, N. 1985. Child labour: A threat to health and development. Defence for Children International, Geneva.
39. Berger, L. R., Belsey, M., Shah, P. M. 1991. Medical aspects of child labor in developing countries. *American Journal of Industrial Medicine* **19**: 697–9.
40. Nersesian, W. S., Petit, M. R., Shaper, R. et al. 1985. Childhood death and poverty: A study of all childhood deaths in Maine, 1976–80. *Pediatrics* **75**: 41–50.
41. Mare, R. D. 1982. Socioeconomic effects on child mortality in the United States. *American Journal of Public Health* **72**: 539–47.
42. Mierley, M. C., Baker, S. P. 1983. Fatal house fires in an urban population. *JAMA* **249**: 1466–8.
43. Rivara, F. P., Barber, M. 1985. Demographic analysis of childhood pedestrian injuries. *Pediatrics* **76**: 375–81.
44. Committee on Trauma Research: Injury in America, National Academy Press, Washington, D.C., 1985.
45. International Society of Child and Adolescent Injury Prevention, C/o CAPT, 4th Floor, Clerks Court, 18–20 Farrington Lane, London EC1R3AU, United Kingdom.

FURTHER READINGS

1. Smith, G. S., Barss, P. 1991. Unintentional injuries in developing countries. The Epidemiology of a neglected problem. *Epidemiologic Reviews* **13**: 228–66.

2. Barss, P., Smith, G. S., Mohan, D., Baker, S. P. 1991. Injuries to adults in developing countries: Epidemiology and policy, The World Bank, Washington, D.C.

3. New approaches to improve road safety: Report of a WHO Study Group. Technical Report Series 781, WHO, Geneva, 1989.

4. Women and health. 1987. *World Health Statistics Quarterly* 40: (3).

5. Vehicle safety in developing countries, WHO, Geneva, 1984. IRP/APR 216m 27B(S).

6. Epidemiology of work-related diseases and accidents. Tenth Report of the Joint ILO/WHO Committee on Occupational Health. Technical Report Series 777, WHO, Geneva, 1989.

7. Improving environmental health conditions in low-income settlements: A community-based approach to identifying needs and priorities. WHO Offset Publication, No. 100, WHO, Geneva, 1987.

2

Injury Information for Action

INJURIES AND ACCIDENTS

An *injury* can be defined as damage to a person caused by an acute transfer of energy, or by a sudden absence of heat (hypothermia) or oxygen (asphyxiation, drowning). Forms of energy are mechanical (kinetic), thermal, chemical, electrical and radiation (Table 2.1). *Intentional injuries* are injuries that are purposefully inflicted, either by the victims themselves (suicide and suicide attempts) or by other persons (homicide, assault, rape, child abuse).

Table 2.1
Injuries as Transfers of Energy

Form of Energy	Examples of Injuries
Mechanical	Fractures
	Lacerations
	Subdurals
Thermal	Heat stroke
	Scald burns
Electrical	Asystole Burns
Chemical	Lead encephalopathy
	Methemoglobinemia from nitrates
	Corneal scars from corrosives
Radiation	Radiation sickness
	Post-irradiation cancers

'Accident' is often used to mean an *event* that produces, or has the potential to produce, an injury. For example, a report from India noted that in 1978, there were 21,500 deaths, and 97,600 persons were injured, as a result of 137,500 road accidents.[1] On the other hand, many articles refer to the number of 'accidents' treated in an emergency department or hospitalized in a certain community. In these articles, the word 'accident' is used synonymously with 'injury,' 'injury victim', or 'casualty'. Problems of translation add to the confusion. In the French language, for example, there is no direct translation of the word 'injuries'. Instead, the words *'les traumatismes'* or *'les accidents'* are used.

Many public health experts believe that widespread use of the term 'accident' has not only caused semantic confusion, it has actually inhibited efforts to reduce injuries.[2, 3] This is because many people think of an 'accident' as being something unpredictable and random, and therefore not preventable. Another connotation of 'accidents' is that they are the result of human carelessness, that the injured person is to blame for his or her injury. In actuality, the events which produce damage to people are non-random, have identifiable risk factors, and involve interactions among people, vehicles, equipment, and processes, and the physical and social environment. As noted in Chapter Six, most injuries are highly preventable through educational, regulatory, and engineering approaches. For these reasons, the word 'accident' is largely avoided in this book.

SOURCES AND LIMITATIONS OF INJURY DATA

Reliable data on injuries are necessary to:

- assess the nature and extent of injuries in a population,
- identify groups that are most at risk for specific injuries,
- establish priorities for intervention,
- allocate appropriate resources for injury control programmes,
- design countermeasures,
- evaluate the effectiveness of laws, technological changes, environmental modifications, and educational campaigns in reducing injuries,
- convince the public and policymakers of the importance of certain injuries and the need for appropriate action.

Summary statistics for cross country comparisons are available from a variety of sources (Table 2.2). Most of these summaries, however, are based on statistics submitted by government agencies within the individual countries. The completeness and reliability of the data can vary widely, as discussed in Chapter One.

Table 2.2
Sources for International Statistics

United Nations Headquarters:
Statistical Yearbook
Demographic Yearbook
Industrial Statistics Yearbook
Population and Vital Statistics Report

Food And Agricultural Organization (FAO):
Monthly Bulletin of Statistics

International Civil Aviation Organization:
Civil Aviation Statistical Yearbook

International Labour Office (ILO):
Yearbook of Labour Statistics

International Monetary Fund (IMF):
International Financial Statistics

UN Educational, Scientific , And Cultural Organization (UNESCO):
Statistical Yearbook

UN Children's Fund (UNICEF):
The State of the World's Children

World Bank:
World Tables – Volume II

World Health Organization (WHO):
World Health Statistics Annual
World Health Statistics Quarterly

Worldwatch Institute:
State of the World Report

Data on injuries within countries are usually quite numerous (Table 2.3). The value and limitations of commonly-used sources of injury information which include death certificates, hospital records, police data, and special surveillance systems are discussed below.

Table 2.3
National Sources of Injury Data

---

1) National registries of deaths (vital statistics)
2) Hospitals and other medical facilities
   - medical records
   - emergency department logs
   - hospital admission or discharge (separation) statistics
   - coroner's and medical examiner's reports
   - poison control center logs
3) Police
   - Motor vehicle events
   - Intentional violence: homicides, assaults, rapes, child abuse, suicides
4) Special surveillance systems
5) Insurance Companies
6) Government Departments (Health, Industry, Police, Mines, Agriculture, etc.)

   Workmen's compensation claims

   Annual reports

   Social service reports on child abuse cases, disability roles

   Special surveys (e.g., national household surveys)
7) Industries and businesses, including transportation companies
8) Judicial system (e.g., Court records of liability claims)
9) Schools (e.g., school health records, school nurse logs)

Vital Statistics Data

Official registries of deaths are often the most accurate source of information on serious injuries occurring in a population. However, in some countries (such as Indonesia), it is legal to cremate or bury the dead without filing a report. Also, mortality data may not be comparable across countries because the persons completing the reports of death may have extensive training (e.g., medical examiners) or none at all (such as untrained village leaders in remote communities).

Hospital Records and Registries

Medical records are vitally important in identifying causes of injury *morbidity* (non-fatal injuries). For example, house fires are the most common cause of burn related deaths; scalds are the most common cause of medically-treated burns. Also, medical records are usually the only source of detailed information about the nature, severity, and costs of all types of injuries in a population. Estimates of the cost of injuries can be based on hospital records of the treatment received, length of stay, and condition of the patient at the time of discharge from the hospital.

Hospital data, however, does have serious limitations:

(i) Patients treated at a individual hospital are often not representative of the total population of injury victims in a community. Geographic, economic, clinical, and other factors result in 'selection bias' when hospital-based, rather than population-based, data is used to analyze injury cases. For example, a hospital with a neurosurgeon on the staff is likely to treat many more patients with head injury than other hospitals. Head injuries may, therefore, appear to be a much more common problem than other injuries in the community. Similarly, private hospitals that cater to upper-income patients are likely to admit more car crash victims than occupationally injured industrial workers. Government hospitals treating poor people in LICs will see more people who are injured as pedestrians and cyclists than as car occupants. A hospital on the outskirts of a city will receive more patients with agricultural injuries than hospitals in the city centre;

(ii) Because it is often not possible to identify the catchment area of a particular hospital, population-based incidence rates cannot be calculated;

(iii) Medical records generally have little or no information on the circumstances of the injury or the occupation of the victim;

(iv) Injuries, such as drownings and pesticide poisonings, that often result in immediate death will be under represented in hospital data. For example, a hospital based study of motorcycle victims may find that 40 per cent of neck injured patients had been wearing a helmet when injured, yet only 20 per cent of riders in the community wear helmets. A wrong conclusion is that helmets double the risk of neck injury. Instead, many more riders without helmets die at the scene from their head and neck injuries. They are therefore not represented in the hospital cases. Unfortunately, once mistaken ideas get established in the public consciousness, it is difficult to counter them.

Police

Police are most often involved when injuries are caused by motor vehicles or intentional violence. Useful epidemiologic data from police reports is often limited like cause of death or injury and the victim's age and sex are often the only variables recorded. Other limitations of police data are:

- many injury events are not reported to the police. For example, a cyclist who is struck by a motor vehicle is often rushed to a hospital without waiting for police to arrive on the scene. In many poor communities, people fear the police and would rather avoid contact with them than report an injury. Also in these communities, well-to-do individuals (such as drivers of automobiles that hit pedestrians) prefer to pay injury victims (or their relatives) to not report injuries, rather than risk large fines or jail terms. Injuries also may be grossly under-reported at times or places where police are scarce (e.g., in rural areas of HICs at night or on the distant islands of Indonesia),
- assessment of injury severity by police is unreliable. A person transported to a hospital usually will be classified as a 'severe' injury, even if he is immediately released with no treatment. A person said to have only 'minor' injuries can subsequently be diagnosed with a ruptured spleen or intracranial haemorrhage,
- assignment of 'cause of accident' by police is heavily influenced by legal concerns (designating a driver at fault). Design and environmental factors (such as road configuration and lighting, vehicle characteristics) may be completely ignored,
- data on alcohol involvement is very unreliable, since it usually depends on a police officer smelling alcohol on a person's breath, and
- special enforcement efforts and campaigns (e.g., to arrest more drunk drivers) can heavily influence police statistics.

Nevertheless, police data can be of considerable value:

- Fatality data, especially for injuries involving public activities like motor vehicle crashes, can be fairly complete in communities with well funded police departments. Even where police resources are limited, mortality figures can be viewed as minimum estimates for the population.
- For motor vehicle crashes, data regarding victim's age and sex, location and time of injury, is often useful for targeting countermeasures,
- Police collect data year after year, making analysis of trends possible,
- Only the police may record deaths that occur outside of hospitals.

SURVEILLANCE

By surveillance is an on-going, systematic programme of data collection and analysis.[4] The purpose of surveillance is to provide information about the incidence and severity of injuries in a population; to identify new problems early, so that adequate interventions can be possible; to determine priorities for action, both in terms of injury problems and high-risk groups; and to help evaluate preventive measures.

Establishment and maintenance of meaningful surveillance programmes, those that contain accurate, comprehensive data, require enormous investments of time, money and personnel. Instead of a surveillance system, a limited time (e.g., one-month) survey of injuries can be conducted as a baseline and then repeated after six months or a year. Repeated, cross-sectional surveys can often provide all the information necessary for setting priorities and targeting interventions. In addition, special areas of interest can be examined more easily. The population census, conducted once every ten years in many countries, is a repetitive cross-sectional survey.

Examples of surveillance programs are hospital registries that record medical data on specific conditions, such as head trauma, spinal cord injuries, or burns. Among the national surveillance systems established at great effort and expense to specifically gather injury data are NEISS (USA), PORS (Netherlands), and HASS (United Kingdom).

Neiss

The National Electronic Injury Surveillance System (NEISS) is a probability sample of hospital emergency departments in the US and its territories. It is used by the US Consumer Product Safety Commission (CPSC) to provide national estimates of the number and severity of injuries associated with consumer products and treated in hospital emergency departments. Also, the system provides a list of names for follow-up investigations. The 5,939 US hospitals having emergency departments and/or emergency visits were stratified by hospital size and ordered by geographic location. Information from a sample of these hospitals and from other sources (such as death certificates and consumer complaints) guide the CPSC in setting priorities for action or in-depth epidemiologic investigation.

The data collection process involves a NEISS coder who reviews emergency department medical records at the end of each day, searching for consumer product-related injuries. The coder transcribes information onto a coding sheet and types the coded data into a teletypewriter at the hospital. During the late night hours, when telephone traffic is low and prices are less expensive, a central computer polls each of the hospital terminals. The computer system edits the data to ensure correct coding and prepares a daily summary for review by CPSC staff.[5]

Fars

The Fatal Accident Reporting System (FARS) was developed by the US National Highway Traffic Safety Administration (NHTSA) to provide data on fatal traffic accidents in the United States. All accidents that involve a motor vehicle travelling on a public road which results in the death of a person within 30 days of the accident are to be reported by states to the FARS. Data are gathered by analysts who are state employees under contract with NHTSA. Analysts obtain data on fatalities for coding on standard forms from police accident reports, vehicle registration files, state driver licensing files, highway department data, death certificates, coroner's and medical examiner's reports, hospitals, and emergency medical services reports.

Each analyst enters the data via a local terminal directly into a central computer. The data are automatically checked for acceptable

Table 2.4

PORS coding form	
PORS	PORS Reference no.
Privé Ongevallen Registratie Systeem (Home and Leisure Accident Surveillance System)	

Coding form

Hospital   `0  6`

AETA*/Patient number   `[          ]`

GP reference   `[    ]`

Date of accident treatment   `[        ]`   `[      ]`

Date of hospital dismissal   `[        ]`   `[    ]`

Follow-up treatment   `[    ]`

Age of patient   `[      ]`

Sex of patient   `[  ]`

Type of accident   `[    ]`

Activity   `[    ]`   if sport: `[      ]`

Location of accident   `[    ]`

Product causing accident   `[        ]`

Product causing injury   `[        ]`

Other product   `[        ]`

Part of body injured   1st `[      ]`   2nd `[      ]`

Type of injury   1st `[      ]`   2nd `[      ]`

How the accident occurred: _____

_____

_____

* to be defined

range values and for consistency. The FARS file contains descriptions of each fatal accident characterizing the accident, the vehicles, and the people involved. Data are available from 1975 to the present. Because FARS data does not include any personal identifying information (such as names or addresses), it is fully available to the public. An annual report highlights the year's data.[6]

Pors

PORS is the acronym for the Home and Leisure Accident Surveillance System of the Netherlands Consumer Safety Institute (CSI). Operational since 1983, PORS records all injuries other than traffic- and occupational-related, treated at 14 participating hospitals. In 1985, the number of such injuries recorded was 72,446. The homes are a representative sample of the 139 general and university teaching hospitals in the country with 24-hour emergency departments. Every 2.5 years, seven of the hospitals are replaced; thus, hospitals participate in PORs project for a maximum of five years. Part-time employees of CSI code all relevant injury cases from medical records. Twice a week the coded forms are mailed to CSI, where the data are checked and then added to the database. The single page coding form (Table 2.4) has a detailed training manual to ensure accuracy of the coded information. The PORS system was a model for EHLASS, the European Home and Leisure Accident Surveillance System established by the European Community.[7]

Hass

The Consumer Safety Unit of the Department of Trade and Industry in the United Kingdom has collected information on home injuries for more than ten years in 20 hospitals in England and Wales through the Home Accident Surveillance System (HASS). Recently, data has been collected on leisure injuries also and hospitals from Scotland and Northern Ireland were also included. A Home Accident Deaths Database (HADD) combines records from several data sources, including manually encoded death registration forms. A new computerized information system was developed to complement HAAS called the Hazardous Products Database. Intended to provide information about potentially hazardous consumer products, the database includes:

- direct consumer complaints,
- voluntary recalls of products by manufacturers,
- warnings to the public about potentially unsafe products,
- results of laboratory tests of suspect products, and
- reports from enforcement authorities about potentially unsafe goods.

PROBLEMS WHEN DATA SYSTEMS ARE NOT LINKED

At times, several different organizations record information about the same injury. Consider a truck driver who dies in the operating room from a head injury after a motor vehicle crash. There may be a form about the crash in the local police files; a medical record at the hospital; an 'accident report' at the truck company; and a death certificate in the vital statistics registry. If the truck driver died at the scene of the crash, however, there would be no medical record. If the driver had no insurance with the truck company, no 'accident report' would necessarily be filed after his death. If the ambulance had to bring the driver to a hospital in a different city, there would be no record of the collision in the local police files. If the physician does not know, or does not record, that the injury occurred while the driver was on-duty for the truck company, the death certificate will not list the fatality as 'occupational-related.' Because the different recording systems, police, hospital, truck company, are not linked, very different injury statistics can be reported for the same type of injury.

Another example involves railway injuries in India:

> Indian Railways (IR) report that there are less than 1,000 fatalities due to railway events every year. Police statistics, on the other hand, show more than 10,000 annual railway deaths. The discrepancy arises because IR only records as 'railway fatalities' those deaths arising from events where a railway employee or railway equipment was at fault. A person falling off a railway carriage or one run over on the railroad tracks is not considered a 'railway fatality'. The police, however, classify as 'railway fatalities' all deaths, even suicides, resulting from an incident involving a train.

INTERPRETING AVAILABLE DATA

Figure 2.1 shows a wide range of burn fatality rates among European countries.[8] Before concluding that economic or cultural differences must account for the variation, it is important to learn more about the statistics from each country. Perhaps some countries had more complete reporting of burns, or included smoke inhalation deaths or

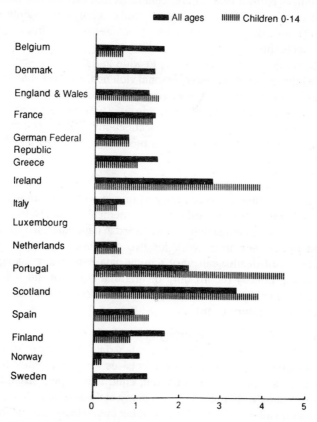

Figure 2.1: Geographic variations in injury rates are well illustrated by data from Europe. The figure shows deaths from fire and flames per 100,000 related population for children aged birth to 14 years and for all ages. From Jackson, H., The epidemiology of children's accidents. In Berfenstam, R., Jackson, H., Eriksson, B. (eds): The Healthy Community: Child Safety as a part of Health Promotion Activities. Stockholm, 1987, p. 43. Folksam Insurance Group, WHO Regional Office for Europe, Child Accident Prevention Trust.

excluded fire-fighters from their data totals. To understand the value and limitations of any summary of injury statistics, several questions are important:

1. What types of injuries were included in the data gathering?

In the category of 'Poisonings', for example, some countries include poisonings from lead, foods, alcohol, illegal drugs, and carbon monoxide; others restrict reporting to chemicals and medicines. 'Burns' may or may not include victims of smoke inhalation. Intentional injuries (homicide, suicide, etc.) are sometimes omitted from statistics on 'accidents.'

Types of injuries that are subject to wide variations among countries are injuries involving interpersonal violence, war and civil strife, suicides, and natural disasters; environmental poisonings (e.g., lead, pesticides, and carbon monoxide); chronic injuries, such as joint disorders from vibration in certain occupations; and miscellaneous categories, such as complications of medical procedures and food poisonings.

2. How were important terms defined?

Police may define a severe injury as one in which an ambulance was called to the scene regardless of the medical diagnosis. In many countries, an occupational injury is included in national statistics only if it led to absence from work for two or more days. Even the enumeration of deaths can vary among data sets. Some agencies (such as the police) record only deaths that occur at the time of reporting. Other data sets include deaths that occur within 30 days or 1 year of the injury event.

3. How complete was the reporting of injuries?

Police statistics, for example, only contain data on injury events for which the police were notified. Even in cases where the police have a .role, such as rape, physical assault, child abuse, pedestrian and cyclist collisions with motor vehicles many of these injury victims go directly to hospitals without the police becoming involved. Hospital statistics will grossly underestimate injuries that result in large numbers of deaths outside the hospital, such as drownings or acute pesticide deaths, and injuries treated in other settings, such as occupational health clinics.

Incomplete reporting is a major problem in any data set that contains a large proportion of the data in categories labelled 'unknown' or 'unspecified'. In one study, for example, death rates from 'Ill-defined causes' ranged from 7.5 per 100,000 population in Sweden to 53.2 in Costa Rica and 360 in El Salvador.[9]

4. What population groups were included?

Data on 'childhood injuries' that include children up to 14 years of age will differ greatly from statistics reporting injuries up to 18 years of age. As noted above, data collected only from hospitals serving poor people will reflect different injury patterns than data that includes reporting from private and military hospitals. The most informative injury data sets are those that capture events from an entire population of individuals, rather than from one or two hospitals. Excellent examples of population-based injury epidemiology involve hospital treated injuries in Ohio, childhood injuries in France and Massachusetts, farm injuries in Sweden and India, and burns in the city of Pittsburgh. The methodologies described in the published papers from these studies are models of injury research.[10-18]

5. What categories were used to summarize the injury data?

Important causes of injury may be lost in summary statistics. Until recently little attention was given to farm-related injuries in children. These injuries were distributed among other categories, motor vehicle, domestic, etc. and therefore were not recognized as a specific problem. Similarly, infants under one year of age were not identified as a special high-risk group for motor vehicle occupant injuries until injury data were plotted by year of age, rather than by age group.[19]

The ranking of injuries as a cause of death will be different in national mortality data that combines all injuries (intentional and unintentional) compared to listings that separate injury causes into motor vehicle, homicide, suicide, and others.

The last section of this chapter has more information about injury classification.

6. What denominators are used to calculate rates?

Fatality rates are often expressed as deaths per 100,000 population. If the population estimates are not accurate or appropriate, the calculated rates will also be inaccurate. For Native American communities in the United States, for example, there are three separate population estimates: from the US Census Bureau, the Indian Health Service, and the Tribes themselves.[20]

Motor-vehicle death rates are often expressed as motor-vehicle related deaths per 10,000 registered vehicles. In some countries, the numbers of vehicles in circulation greatly exceeds the number that are officially registered. This would falsely *increase* the calculated rate.

Often, the most meaningful rates are those based on estimates of exposure to injury risk. For example, sex differences in cycle injury rates disappear when the denominator becomes hours of bicycle use (see 'Female/Male Differences' in Chapter Five). Unfortunately, exposure data is difficult and expensive to collect and therefore rarely available.

One exception in many countries is the availability of 'vehicle kilometres' ('vehicle-miles') data, estimates of the miles travelled by particular vehicles. When the average occupancy of the vehicles is also known, 'person-vehicle-kilometres travelled' can also be used as a denominator for calculating motor vehicle injury rates.[21]

CLASSIFICATION OF INJURIES

Little progress would be made in cancer research, prevention, or treatment if data on cancers were not organized by type of cell, presence of metastases, functional activity, and so on. Similarly, data on injuries are of little value unless they are organized and classified in a way that is informative. Table 2.5 lists *some* of the dimensions under which injuries may be classified. Further detail could be provided within each dimension, such as specifying the particular occupation in a work-related injury. Other dimensions could be added, such as 'involvement of alcohol' or 'consumer product-related'.

Table 2.5
Dimensions for Classifying Injuries

External Causes (Mechanisms) of Injury:

Motor vehicle-related events.
Falls and jumps.
Drowning/submersion.
Other threats to breathing.
Burns.
Poisoning.
Exposure to inanimate mechanical forces.

Exposure to animate mechanical force.
Exposure to other natural and environmental factors.
Complications or misadventures involving medical and surgical care.
Other and unknown.

Intent:

Accidental/unintentional.
Assault/intentional violence.
Self-inflicted.
Legal intervention or operation of war.
Unspecified or unknown intent.

Nature of Injury:

Fracture.
Concussion.
Internal bleeding.
Laceration.
Other.

Body Part(s) Involved:

Skull, chest, abdomen, extremities, etc.

Site or Place of Occurrence:

Traffic area: motorways, highways, roads, streets, etc.
Residential area: residences, including access roads, yards, footpaths,
    garages.
Industrial/workshop area: factories, power plants, buildings under
    construction, etc.
Trade and service area open to the public: shops, supermarkets,
    warehouses, etc.
Farm.
Schools.
Residential institutions and public administrative areas.
Sports and athletic area: swimming baths, gymnasiums, and athletic
    grounds, etc.
Public entertainment and park area: restaurants, pubs, cinema and
    concert halls.

Other outdoor area: mountains, uncultivated lands, woods, beaches, rivers, etc.

Other specified area.

Unspecified or unknown area.

Activity of the Victim at the Time of Injury:

Engaged in work (occupational injury).

Attending school.

Engaged in sports or recreation.

Performing housework.

Performing some other activity.

Unknown.

There is no single, correct way to classify injuries. Any classification will have value only in relation to the purpose (or purposes) for which it is to be used. If a surgeon wants information on patient injuries associated with poor outcomes, more detailed clinical categories would be necessary. Similarly, traffic police, occupational health experts, and consumer safety advocates all have different information needs. For the purpose of injury prevention, the single most important dimension is listed first in Table 2.5: the mechanism (external cause) of injury. Many agencies collect statistics about injuries categorized solely by 'nature of injury' (fractures, lacerations, head trauma, etc.). With this data, there is no way of knowing whether the fractures were caused by falls or motor vehicles/pedestrian collisions, whether the head trauma was a result of assaults or motorcycles.

The categories in any classification scheme should be exhaustive, meaning that no possibilities are omitted, and mutually exclusive—meaning that it should not be possible to include a case in more than one category. This is no simple task. Consider a scheme that classifies injuries into four categories: occupational, motor-vehicle, intentional, and other/non-intentional (e.g., sports and domestic injuries). That these categories are over-lapping (not mutually exclusive) is illustrated by a hypothetical example: Robbers escaping from a bank purposefully drive their car into a police officer, causing a femoral fracture. In the proposed scheme, the policeman's injury would fit into *three* categories: motor vehicle, occupational, and intentional. A real example arises from a study of 138 workers who died from work-related injuries during a one-year period in Maryland.[22] Forty-one per cent of the deaths involved transportation vehicles. An additional 16 per cent involved non-road land vehicles. In other words, more than half the *occupational* deaths were *motor-vehicle* related.

Both *intentional* and *unintentional* injuries are vital to include in any comprehensive survey of injuries in a community. Admittedly, it is sometimes very difficult to classify a particular injury according to *intent*. A person who drowns may have been swept away by a strong current, or may have committed suicide. A woman who dies from burns in India may have been the victim of a cooking fire, marital discord, or of a conflict over her dowry. A twelve year-old boy who kills a ten year-old companion with a handgun may have fired the weapon accidentally, or with the conscious purpose of eliminating a competitor in the cocaine market. A toddler with a scald burn on her legs may have burned herself in very hot bath water, or may have been burned as punishment by an angry parent.

Despite these difficulties, intent is an extremely important dimension from a preventive standpoint. For example, a review of death certificates of 348 cases of fatal occupational injuries to civilian females in Texas (1975–1984) found that homicides accounted for 53 per cent.[23] Strategies to prevent these deaths would have to address intentional violence as a priority. Similarly, in Thailand in 1983, the homicide death rate (16.6 per 100,000 population) exceeded the death rate from motor vehicles (13.3 per 100,000) and tuberculosis (11.2 per 100,000).[24]

A major problem for any classification system is that medical records often lack sufficient information to assign appropriate categories. For example, what the injury control specialist would like to see in the medical record is: 'Seventeen year old white female presents with 6 centimeter laceration of right hand with tendon damage after tripping and falling through a plate glass window at school.' What the medical record is likely to say is: 'Hand lac'.[25]

INTERNATIONAL INJURY CLASSIFICATION

The most widely used system for classification of diagnoses is the World Health Organization's 'International Statistical Classification of Diseases and Related Health Problems', abbreviated as 'ICD'. The

Tenth Revision (ICD–10), published in English and French, was released in 1993.[26]

The classification of injuries in 'ICD–10' is a radical departure from 'ICD–9', the current revision. In 'ICD–9', injuries are classified according to the *type of injury* (fracture, burn, laceration) and *site of injury* (skull, trunk, abdomen, etc.). A separate set of codes (E codes) appear as a supplement to the main classification. The 'E codes' are used to further classify injuries by External Cause, i.e., *mechanisms of injury.* For example, E800 refers to 'Railway accident involving collision with rolling stock' and E999 to 'Late effect of injury due to war operations.'[27]

In 'ICD–10', there are again two primary sets of codes for injury: 'External Causes of Morbidity and Mortality' (Chapter XX, letters V–Y) and types of injury (listed under letters S and T in Chapter XIX, 'Injury, Poisoning and Certain Other Consequences of External Causes'). For example, injuries to the thorax are coded S20–S29, burns and corrosions are T20–T32. The short list for injury-related deaths by external cause is as follows:

Transport accidents	V00–V99
Falls	W00–W19
Accidental drowning	W65–W74
Exposure to smoke, fire and flames	X00–X09
Accidental poisoning by and exposure to noxious substances	X40–X49
Intentional self-harm (suicide)	X60–X84
Assault	X85–Y09
All other external causes	W20–W64, W75–W99, X10–X39, X50–X57, Y10–Y89.

Causes of death should be tabulated according to both Chapter XIX (type of injury) and Chapter XX (External Cause) codes. If only one code is tabulated, the external cause code should be used in preference to the Chapter XIX code.

With ICD–10, it is possible, by adding supplementary digits, to code for 'Activity at the time of injury' (sports, leisure, working for income, etc.). There is also opportunity for coding supplementary factors that contribute to injury. For example, Y90 is 'Evidence of alcohol with involvement determined by blood alcohol content'.

Two separate but wholly comparable versions of ICD–10 will be issued: one with three-character categories and another with four-character categories. This will enable countries with widely different data needs and resources to utilize the same classification scheme. The following is an example of how an injury event would be coded in the ICD–10 classification scheme:

> While driving his motorcycle to the scene of an emergency, a police officer was struck by a van. He died from a massive head injury. The blood alcohol level of the van's driver (who was not seriously injured) was 220 mg/100 ml; the police officer's blood alcohol level was 0 mg/100 ml.

External Cause of Death

V23.42–Motorcycle driver injured in a collision with a car, pickup truck, or van in a traffic accident occurring while working for income.

Type of Injury

S07.1–Crushing injury of skull.

Supplementary Factors

Y90.0–Blood alcohol level of less than 20 mg/100 ml.

Note that the high blood alcohol level of the van's driver is *not* captured by the ICD–10 scheme. This, and other possible limitations of the new classification system will undoubtedly be discussed before WHO issues ICD–11.

SEVERITY

Country X passes a law requiring motorcyclists to wear helmets. One year later, statistics show that more victims of motorcycle crashes are being treated in emergency rooms, although the number of motorcycles on the road has not changed.

Does this mean that helmets increase the risk of injury?

Country Y reports a rate of burn injuries of 16 per million population.

Adjacent Country Z, whose population is similar in age distribution and economic status, reports a rate of 160 per million.

Could the ten-fold difference in rates be due to a statistical error?

City D invests $100,000 to train ambulance drivers in advanced resuscitation techniques. Although the mortality rate of motor vehicle victims remains unchanged in City D, the average time of transport from the crash site to the hospital increased by 2 minutes.

Was the money wasted?

To answer any of the questions requires a knowledge of injury severity. Rating severity is vital when comparing injury rates across populations and over time; making assessments about the prognosis of injured patients; evaluating pre-hospital and in-hospital care; or determining the effectiveness of products and interventions to reduce injuries.

A major reason for recording injury severity is that the most common causes of severe injuries are usually not the most common causes of less-severe injuries. In most industrialized countries, for example, scald burns are the most common type of burn to children treated in out-patient settings. House fires, not scalds, are the most common cause of death from burns in childhood. Similarly, motor-vehicle injuries are the number one cause of death in children and young adults in many countries. However, falls, burns, and poisonings are more common reasons for emergency department visits.

Classifying injuries by whether the victim died, was admitted to a hospital, or was treated on an out-patient basis and released is a simple, but powerful, approach to severity rating (or scaling). This approach is adequate for many purposes in populations where access to health care is widespread. In LICs, however, many individuals with severe injuries never receive any form of medical attention. In these countries, a comprehensive picture of the extent of injuries of all severity can only be obtained by household surveys.

More elaborate schemes for scaling severity of injury take different approaches. Some schemes consider an injury severe if it has severe immediate effects (e.g., loss of consciousness, compound fracture, multiple injuries); if the outcome for the patient is serious (death, permanent disability or disfigurement); if the resources required for treatment are great (e.g., surgery, invasive diagnostic tests); if there is a serious threat to life; or if it takes a long time to recover from the injury.

Specific types of injuries have unique aspects to consider in relation to severity. An injury to the head, for example, will have anatomic (depressed skull fracture), physiologic (papilloedema, abnormal pupillary responses) and functional impacts (e.g., the Glasgow Coma Scale assigns scores for eye opening, motor, and verbal responses).[28] Assessment of burn severity includes estimation of the surface area burned, the depth of burn, and the parts of the body involved (a third degree burn involving the face has more serious consequences than one involving the same surface area of the leg).[29] Even the age and sex of the patient influences the severity of an injury: a chest burn will be more devastating for a girl than for a boy; an infant who is vigorously shaken by an angry adult may suffer an intracranial haemorrhage, while a teenager will be unharmed.

Estimates of the number of injury-related hospitalizations or emergency visits in a population are often made by multiplying the number of injury deaths by a constant. This approach is based on the assumption that a fixed ratio exists among injury-related deaths, hospitalizations, and emergency visits: 'For every person killed in motor vehicle crashes, y number are admitted to hospitals and z number are seen in emergency rooms.' The assumption of fixed ratios can be very misleading, as data from the Netherlands illustrates (Table 2.6).[30] For injury victims in that country, the overall ratio of deaths to hospitalizations to 'other medical treatment' is 1:20:493. In other words, for each injury victim who died, there were 20 people hospitalized and almost 500 who received some form of medical treatment for their injury. For industrial injuries, however, the ratio becomes 1:175:938; for traffic injuries, 1:11:16, and for home injuries, 1:23:917!

Table 2.6
Injuries in the Netherlands, 1980

Category of injuries	Fatal	Hospital Admissions	Other Medical Treatment
Industrial	80	14,000	75,000
Traffic	2,200	24,000	35,000
Home and leisure	2,400	55,000	2,200,000
Total	4,680	93,000	2,310,000

Abbreviated Injury Scale (AIS) and
Injury Severity Score (ISS)

The scaling system most commonly used in studies of motor vehicle and other types of injuries is the AIS.[31, 32] With this scale, each injury is categorized by *body area* and *severity*. There are separate AIS scores for typical injuries to seven major body areas (AIS scores for chest injuries are outlined in Table 2.7). AIS scores range from 1 (minor injury) to 6 (maximum injury—survival unprecedented). AIS 6 injuries would include a massively crushed head or transected torso.

Table 2.7
The Abbreviated Injury Scale (AIS): Codes for Chest Injuries

AIS CODE	INJURY DESCRIPTION
1. Minor	Muscle ache or chest wall stiffness.
2. Moderate	Simple rib or sternal fractures; major contusions of chest wall without hemothorax or pneumothorax or respiratory embarrassment.
3. Serious, not life-threatening	Multiple rib fractures without respiratory embarrassment; hemothorax or pneumothorax; rupture of diaphragm; lung contusion.
4. Severe, life-threatening, survival probable	Open chest wounds; frail chest; pneumomediastinum; myocardial contusion without circulatory embarrassment; pericardial injuries.
5. Critical, survival uncertain	Chest injuries with major respiratory embarrassment (laceration of trachea, hemomediastinum, etc.); aortic laceration; myocardial rupture or contusion with circulatory embarrassment.
6. Maximum injury, virtually unsurvivable	Transection of torso.

The AIS pertains to individual injuries. Most deaths following auto-motive crashes involve injury to more than one part of the body. It is therefore not surprising that the AIS rating for the most severe injury does not correlate well with mortality rates. To achieve a better correlation, the Injury Severity Score (ISS) was derived.[33, 34] First, each injury is separately rated with the AIS. The sum of the squares of the three highest separate AIS scores yields the ISS (Table 2.8).[35]

Table 2.8
Calculating an Injury Severity Score

Case: An 18-year-old man in motor vehicle accident with multiple injuries

Body region	Nature of injuries	AIS	$(AIS)^2$
External	Contusions, chest, abdomen and extremities	2	4
Head	Closed head injury, unspecified	2	–
Face	Lip laceration	1	–
Chest	Right pneumothorax	3	9
Abdomen	Spleen laceration	4	16
Extremities	Fracture clavicle	2	–
	ISS =	–	29

The ISS performs much less well as a predictor of disability, as opposed to mortality. One reason is that the specific *body region of the most severe injury sustained* has a powerful impact on subsequent disability. Injuries to the head and spine are most likely to result in disability; abdominal and thoracic injuries, if the patient survives, usually have no long-term sequence.

A study was made of 266 persons who were hospitalized for trauma. All had been working full-time prior to injury. Within the first month post-injury, only 19 per cent of those with moderate/severe extremity injuries, 13 per cent of those with severe head/neck injuries, and 7 per cent of those with a spinal cord injury had returned to work. Nearly 40 per cent of the individuals without these injuries were employed at one month.[36]

The AIS and its derivative, ISS, were devised for studies of motor vehicle injuries. They do not work equally well for other types of trauma, such as poisonings, gun shots, or electrical injuries. Overall, severity scales have most value in analyzing data from groups of injury victims. Their usefulness in predicting the outcome of individual injury victims is limited.

ECONOMIC COSTS OF INJURIES

The importance of injuries is also reflected in economic costs to the individual victim and family, to the medical care system, and to society. Cost-analysis has assumed increasing importance in policy making at all levels of government. Many of the techniques for estimating costs were developed to justify expensive construction projects. Today, estimates of the financial impact of decisions, including public health and medical programs, are usually a requirement for planning. Obviously, methods that are appropriate for analyzing the costs and benefits of a dam cannot be easily adapted to estimating the cost of a population-based health education effort or a law requiring motorcycle riders to wear helmets. Consider a government regulation that would require placing a rear-view mirror on the right side of all automobiles sold in a country. Although the mirror would cost only $10 to install, the 1 million vehicles sold each year would mean a total expense of $10 million. Let us say that the mirror would result in fewer motor vehicle crashes, saving 10 lives and preventing 100 injuries requiring hospitalization. How would an economist estimate the costs and benefits of such a regulation?

One stumbling block obviously involves placing a value on a human life. Among the approaches that have been used are:

— estimating lifetime earnings,
— relying on past social policy decisions,
— using court awards in cases of wrongful death,
— reviewing life insurance policies for amounts of coverage, and
— administering questionnaires that ask persons to state how much they would be willing to pay for certain reductions in risk.

All of these approaches have serious limitations, practically and conceptually. For example, the amount of life insurance a person buys is much more related to the family's financial needs than to how much a person values his or her own life.

Even gathering data on the most easily measurable costs, the so-called 'direct costs' such as hospital and physician charges, medications, and transportation, is difficult. The list of direct costs is extensive (Table 2.9)[37] and the information is not always recorded in a useable form.

Table 2.9
Partial List of Direct Costs

Emergency services: Ambulance, emergency room, personnel (emergency medical technician/paramedics, physicians, nurses, etc.), blood bank, medications.

Hospital inpatient costs: Services, physicians, operating room, drugs.

Hospital outpatient department: Services, medications, appliances.

Office-based: physicians and nurses.

Rehabilitation: Physical, occupational, speech and hearing therapy, prostheses.

Long-term care: Custodial care, modification of home environment (e.g., wheelchair ramps).

Home-health services: Nurse, aides, homemakers.

Administrative costs: Insurance companies, government medical agencies; vehicle, barrier, and other property damage.

Legal fees and court costs.

Police costs.

Welfare and human services costs: Social worker, medical social worker, support payments.

Funeral and medical examiner costs.

Costs for other affected persons: Witnesses' time in court, family members.

'Indirect costs' include earnings that are lost as a result of death or disability; the value of time, production, and consumption lost because family members must care for the accident victim; and the 'costs' associated with suffering and disfigurement. The difficulty (and arbitrariness) of estimating such costs are obvious.

Estimating the economic costs of injuries is even more problematic in LICs. Should the negligible wages workers receive, be used to calculate the economic cost of a labourer's death, or should some estimate be made of the 'real' value of his labour? When social support systems (workmen's compensation, food supplement programmes, government-sponsored health care) are virtually non-existent, serious injury or death of a wage earner can devastate a poor family in an LIC. How can this be reflected in economic calculations? In a landmark judgement in India, the Supreme Court ruled that compensation for victims of industrial injuries would depend on the corporation's ability to pay, rather than on the previous income of the victim.

In countries where hospitals are heavily subsidized by the government, the fees charged to patients are a fraction of the actual expenses. The cost of care to the nation, rather than to the individual, is therefore a more accurate reflection of true medical costs.

Much of the economic impact of injuries simply cannot be measured. What is the cost to a country of having six of its physicians killed in a car crash when the ratio of doctors to population is one to 300,000? What is the loss when a pianist has a finger amputated by a defective household appliance? Statistics on health-care costs can only hint at the magnitude of the problem.

A method of economic decision making that avoids some of the above problems is called 'cost-effectiveness analysis' (CEA). CEA begins with a specific objective such as like reducing motor vehicle deaths and compares the costs of different programmes proposed to reach that objective. For example, Programme A costs $100,000 and would save 2 lives; Programme B costs $200,000 but would save 10 lives. Since Programme A costs $50,000 per life saved and Programme B $20,000, Programme B is more 'cost-effective.' Although CEA avoids the problem of assigning monetary values to everything, it has its own serious limitations. For one thing, is it often very difficult to estimate how effective a programme will be before it is actually implemented. Also, no programme has only one effect; CEA has no means of balancing multiple simultaneous and conflicting outcomes.

The conclusion is not that estimates of costs are completely without value. Rather, cost-analysis must be viewed with some skepticism and humility. It must be one part of a comprehensive approach to injury control that also weighs ethical, social, political, and legal considerations.[38, 39]

REFERENCES

1. Road user cost study in India: Final Report. 1982, Central Road Research Institute, New Delhi.

2. Haddon, W., Baker, S. P. 1981. Injury Control. In: Clark, D. W., Mac-Mahon, B. (eds), Preventive and Community Medicine, Little-Brown and Company, Boston.
3. Robertson, L. S. 1983. Injuries: Causes, Control Strategies, and Public Policy. Lexington Books, D.C. Heath and Company, Lexington.
4. Graitcer, P. L. 1987. The development of state and local injury surveillance systems. *Journal of Safety Research* 18: 191–8.
5. Division of Hazard and Injury Data Systems, US Consumer Product Safety Commission: The NEISS Sample–Design and Implementation. March, 1986.
6. Fatal Accident Reporting System Yearly Report. Available from the National Highway Traffic Safety Administration, 400, 7th Street SW, Washington, D.C., 20590, USA.
7. Mulder, S. (PORS) 1986. Annual Review of the Home and Leisure Accident Surveillance System. Consumer Safety Institute, Amsterdam.
8. Jackson, H. 1987. The epidemiology of children's accidents. In: Berfenstam, R., Jackson, H., Eriksson, B. (eds), The Healthy Community: Child Safety as a part of Health Promotion Activities, Folksam Insurance Company, Stockholm, Sweden, p. 43.
9. Baker, T. 1977. Assessment of health status and needs. International Health Perspectives, Volume 2, Springer Publishing Company, New York, p. 9.
10. Barancik, J. I., Chatterjee, B. F., Greene, Y. C. et al. 1983. Northeast Ohio Trauma Study: I. Magnitude of the problem. *American Journal of Public Health* 73: 746–51.
11. Fife, D., Barancik, J. I., Chatterjee, B. F. 1984. Northeast Ohio Trauma Study: II. Injury rates by age, sex, and cause. *American Journal of Public Health* 74: 473–8.
12. Tiret, L., Garros, B., Maurette, P. et al. 1989. Incidence, causes, and severity of injuries in Aquitaine, France: A community-based study of hospital admissions and deaths. *American Journal of Public Health* 79: 316–21.
13. Tursz, A. 1991. Collection of data on accidents in childhood. In: Manciaux, M., Romer, C. J. (eds), *Accidents in Childhood and Adolescence: The Role of Research*, WHO, Geneva.
14. Tursz, A., Crost, M., Guyot, M. et al. 1985. Childhood accidents: a registration in public and private medical facilities of a French health care area. *Public Health* 99: 154–64.
15. Gallagher, S. S., Guery, B., Kotelchuck, M. et al. 1982. A strategy for the reduction of childhood injuries in Massachusetts: SCIPP. *New England Journal of Medicine* 307: 1015–19.
16. Jansson, B. 1988. Agriculture and Injuries: A System for Injury Surveillance in Swedish Emergency Care as a Basis of Injury Control, FOLKSAM/Karolinska Institute, Sundbyberg, Sweden.

17. Barancik, J. I., Shapiro, M. A. 1975. Pittsburgh burn study. Report No. PB 250–737. National Technical Information Service, Springfield, Virginia.
18. Varghese, M., Mohan, D. 1990. Occupational Injuries among Agricultural Workers in Rural Haryana, India. *Journal of Occupational Accidents* 12: 237–44.
19. Baker, S. P. 1979. Motor vehicle occupant deaths in young children. *Pediatrics* 64: 860–1.
20. Berger, L. R., Kitzes, J. 1989. Injuries to children in a native American community. *Pediatrics* 84: 152–6.
21. Bangdiwala, S. I., Anzola-Perez, E., Glizer, I. M. 1985. Statistical considerations for the interpretation of commonly utilized road traffic accident indicators: Implications for developing countries. *Accident Analysis and Prevention* 17: 419–27.
22. Baker, S. P., Samkoff, J. S., Fisher, R. S. et al. 1982. Fatal occupational injuries. *Journal of the American Medical Association* 248: 692–7.
23. Davis, H., Honchar, P. A., Suarez, L. 1987. Fatal occupational injuries of women, Texas 1975–1984. *American Journal of Public Health* 77: 1524–7.
24. Kanchanaraksa, S. 1987. Review of the health situation in Thailand: Priority ranking of diseases. National Epidemiology Board of Thailand, Bangkok.
25. Berenholz, G., Azzara, C. A., Gallagher, S. S. 1985. The medical record as a source document in injury surveillance systems. APHA Meeting, Washington, D.C., November 18.
26. ICD-10: International Statistical Classification of Diseases and Related Health Problems. Tenth Revision, World Health Organization, Geneva, 1992.
27. The International Classification of Diseases, Ninth Revision (ICD-9), World Health Organization, Geneva, 1979.
28. Jennett, B., Teasdale, G., Galbraith, S. et al. 1977. Severe head injuries in three countries. *J Neurol Neurosurg Psychol* 40: 291.
29. Sanderson, L. M., Buffler, P. A., Perry, R. R. et al. 1981. A multi-variate evaluation of determinants of length of stay in a hospital burn unit. *Journal of Burn Care and Rehabilitation* 2: 142–9.
30. About home and leisure accidents, and their prevention in the Netherlands, Consumer Safety Institute, Amsterdam, 1982.
31. AMA Committee on Medical Aspects of Automotive Safety. 1971. Rating the Severity of Tissue Damage. I. The Abbreviated Scale. *JAMA* 215: 277–80.
32. The Abbreviated Injury Scale, 1990 Revision. American Association for Automotive Medicine, Des Plaines, Illinois 60018, USA.
33. Baker, S. P., O'Neill, B., Haddon, W., Long, W. B. 1974. The Injury Severity Score: A method for describing patients with multiple injuries and evaluating emergency care. *Journal of Trauma* 14: 187–96.

34. Baker, S. P., O'Neill, B. 1976. The Injury Severity Score: An update. *Journal of Trauma* **16**: 882–5.
35. Smith, N. 1987. The incidence of severe trauma in small rural hospitals. *Journal of Family Practice* **25**: 595–600.
36. MacKenzie, E. J., Shapiro, S., Smith, R. T. et al. 1987. Factors influencing return to work following hospitalization for traumatic injury. *American Journal of Public Health* **77**: 329–34.
37. Berger, L. R. 1981. Childhood injuries: Recognition and prevention. *Current Problems in Pediatrics* **12**: 1–59.
38. Rice, D. P., Mackenzie, E. J. and Associates. 1989. Cost of Injury in the United States: A Report to Congress, Institute for Health and Aging, University of California and Injury Prevention Center, The John Hopkins University, San Francisco, CA.
39. Creese, A., Parker, D. 1990. Cost Analysis in Primary Health Care: A Training Manual for Programme Managers, WHO, Geneva.

FURTHER READINGS

1. Abelin, T., Brzezinski, Z. J., Carstairs, V. D. L. (eds). 1987. Measurement in health promotion and protection. WHO Regional Publications, European Series, No. 22, WHO, Copenhagen.
2. Accidents in children and young people. 1986. *World Health Statistics Quarterly* **39**.
3. Injury Mortality Atlas of the United States, 1979–1987. Centers for Disease Control, Atlanta, Georgia, 1993.
4. Mills, A. 1985. Economic evaluation of health programmes: application of the principles in developing countries. *World Health Statistics Quarterly* **38**.
5. Warner, K. E., Luce, B. R. 1982. Cost-Benefit and Cost-Effectiveness Analysis in Health Care. Health Administration Press, University of Michigan School of Public Health, Ann Arbor, Michigan.

3

Conducting Epidemiological
Research in Injury Control

Unlike clinical medicine, which focuses on individuals, epidemiology concerns itself with populations or groups of individuals. In the area of injuries, epidemiologic methods can help find answers to such questions as:

- What are the most common types of injuries in different age groups?
- What are the characteristics of persons who are most likely to be injured (risk factors and high risk groups)?
- What are the circumstances under which injuries are most likely to occur?
- What policies and programmes can reduce the likelihood and severity of injuries in a community?

SIMPLE APPROACHES TO DATA COLLECTION

Injury studies do not have to be complicated or expensive. Field observations, interviews with key informants, and newspaper content analyses are some of the low-tech, low-cost, and potentially high yield research activities that can shed a great deal of light on injury problems.

An example of a field observation study involved motorcycle helmet use in Bangkok, Thailand:

> The researcher wanted to study helmet use for two reasons: to highlight the need for a comprehensive helmet law; and to obtain baseline data from which the impact of a future helmet law could be assessed.

The study involved standing on a busy street corner, observing riders and passengers on two-wheeled vehicles with and without helmets. The data, collected in one hour, is summarized in Table 3.1. Conclusions from the study were that: there are no major differences between motorcycles and motor-scooters in the proportion of drivers or passengers wearing helmets; drivers are much more likely to be wearing a helmet than passengers (43 per cent vs. 3 per cent); drivers of vehicles without passengers are more than twice as likely to wear helmets as drivers carrying passengers (48 per cent vs. 21 per cent). Recommendations were that a helmet law should cover all motorized two-wheeled vehicles and both drivers and passengers should be required to wear helmets.

Table 3.1

Observations of 405 Motorized Two-wheeled Vehicles at a Bangkok Street Corner, 20 March 1987

	Motorcycles	Motor Scooters
Total number of vehicles observed	305	100
Per cent of drivers wearing helmets	44	41
Per cent of passengers wearing helmets	2 (1/46)	5 (1/21)
Total no. of vehicles with no passengers	260	79
Per cent of drivers wearing helmets	48	47
Total no. vehicles with passengers	45*	21
Per cent of drivers wearing helmets	22 (10/45)	19 (4/21)
Per cent of passengers wearing helmets	2 (1/46)	5 (1/21)

Note: * One motorcycle was carrying a driver with two passengers.

Key informants are individuals who have insights about injury problems because of their in-depth knowledge of a community, day-to-day involvement with injury-related activities, or special expertise. To become acquainted with important injury issues in an isolated rural community in Thailand, for example, a researcher might interview long time residents of the community, practicing physicians, village health workers, police officers, and ambulance drivers (Table 3.2). The list generated by the group can serve as a foundation for designing survey forms or identifying additional sources of data.

An example of a *newspaper content analysis* involved a review of the 'Bangladesh Times:'

Bangladesh has a population of 97 million (1984), a land area of 144,000

Table 3.2

Injury Problems in a Rural Community Cited by a
Group of Key Informants

Burns from farming practices.
Drownings in irrigation canals.
Motor vehicle crashes involving locally made pick up trucks.
Electrocutions from recent electrification projects.
Pesticide poisonings: occupational and suicidal.
Snake and animal bites.
Burns from LPG gas explosions as LPG replaces charcoal.
Falls.
Motorcycle crashes.
Homicides and assaults.
Pedestrian injuries.
Overturning buses.

---

square kilometres, and a sub-tropical monsoon climate. Major industries are jute, sugar, paper, textiles, leather, and fertilizers. The
1985 per capita income was US $163. A national system of death
certificate reporting was not in place in Bangladesh in 1986. To identify
the most common causes of death from injuries, articles from the
Bangladesh Times about injury related deaths were tabulated during
a seven-day period in February, 1986. The importance of intentional
injuries (both suicide and inflicted violence) and motor-vehicles injuries became obvious (Table 3.3).

Table 3.3

One-week's Reports of Injury related Deaths
(Bangladesh Times, February, 1986)

Cause of Reported Death	Number
Violence inflicted by others	16
Suicide	16
Motor vehicle	22
Pedestrian hit by bus or truck	9
Bus, single vehicle	6
Collision of 2 motor vehicles	3
Other motor vehicle	6
Food poisoning	6
All other injury related	5

Of course, a newspaper content analysis has several weaknesses. First, injuries from violence are much more likely to be reported than other deaths because such stories sell newspapers. Second, deaths occurring in cities are more likely to be covered than those in rural areas, simply because reporters are usually not present outside large metropolitan areas. Thus, agricultural injuries involving pesticides and machinery are often missed. Third, less frequent but large-scale causes of injuries (such as the bus that plunged into a river at a ferry terminal the previous week) may not appear during a time-limited (one week or one month) review of the papers. Similarly, seasonal injuries like deaths from flooding during the monsoon season will not appear if injuries are only recorded during the dry season. Nevertheless, newspapers can be a useful source of information when other data systems do not exist or when such systems lack details about the circumstances of injury.[1]

COMPARISON GROUPS

A researcher finds that 25 per cent of working children in a certain community suffer from elevated lead levels. She suspects that child labour is responsible until she discovers that 25 per cent of non-working children of the same age also have high lead levels in their blood. The non-working children illustrate how a comparison group is important in judging the relevance of a finding.

Ideally, individuals in the target and comparison groups should be exactly alike except for the variable of interest (in this case, whether they are working or not). Differences in outcomes between the two groups can then be ascribed solely to the work situation. Obviously, no two groups of individuals can be exactly alike. However, not all differences among people—in hair and eye colour, for example will affect the outcome being studied. Three variables that are important to examine in virtually every study of injuries are *age*, *sex*, and *socioeconomic status*. Consider a study of injuries among students at a local university. You find that the rate of injuries treated in emergency rooms is twice as high as that of the local community. You are about to conclude that there is a serious injury problem at the university until you realize that there may be other explanations:

- The average age of the students at the university is 20 years and that of the general community, 38 years.

- The university only admits males, who in general have a higher rate of injury than females.
- Most of the university students come from well-to-do families. Many of them own cars and motorcycles and all have a health insurance plan that pays for emergency room visits.
- Instead of comparing the students injury rate to that of the local community as a whole, a more appropriate comparison group would be same-aged males from similar socio-economic backgrounds who do not attend the university.

TYPES OF EPIDEMIOLOGICAL STUDIES

The three most common types of epidemiologic studies are *case-control, cohort,* and *cross-sectional* studies. In a *case-control study,* the researcher identifies persons with a specific injury or condition (the outcome) and selects a comparison group consisting of persons without the injury. The proportion of each group with evidence of a particular *exposure* (for example, having worked in a specific occupation) is then compared. Case-control studies are valuable when the injury is infrequent:

> A researcher wants to determine if a diet low in calcium predisposes elderly women to hip fractures from falls. A case-control study is conducted. The 'cases' are elderly women with hip fractures. The 'controls' are women of the same age without fractures. Dietary histories show that the cases report significantly less calcium intake than the controls.

The example illustrates a few of the weaknesses of case-control studies. First, the measure of exposure, dietary histories of calcium intake, are unreliable because they rely on recall. Second, the cases and controls, although of the same age, may differ in important ways. For example, the women with hip fractures may have other illnesses that suppressed their appetite. The association of fractures with low calcium, then, is confounded by poor general nutrition and co-existing illness.

Cohort studies begin with persons whom the researcher knows do *not* have a specific injury or condition. The target individuals are people who have a particular exposure which the comparison individuals do not.

Suspicion that exposure to medical x-rays might contribute to the development of cancer led to a cohort study of physicians. Radiologists were compared to other physicians who did not regularly work with x-ray machines. Death rates from cancer were much higher in the radiologists.

In a cohort study, the temporal sequence of exposure and outcome can be assured, it is possible to make ongoing measurements of exposure (e.g., levels of radiation in the x-ray room or asbestos at a shipyard), and data can be collected on many different exposures and outcomes.

Cohort studies are generally not used when the outcomes are rare or if they occur long after exposure (long latency health effects). Under these circumstances, a cohort study may not detect them even if very large numbers of people are included and followed for many years:

> A hypothetical cohort study is undertaken to determine the risk of leukemia in persons who work in a chemical industry where radioactive chemicals are used. The 3-year study involves 100 chemical workers and 100 workers from other industries. Assuming the risk of leukemia is one case per 3,000 persons per year in the general population, and *ten times* as great in the chemical industry (10 cases per 3,000 workers per year). During the study, we would expect to find only a single case of leukaemia in the working group and none in the comparison group, clearly too few cases to make any scientific conclusions.

Another difficulty of cohort studies is that individuals are likely to 'drop out' before the study is completed for reasons such as changing jobs or moving to another town. For example, if a cohort study begins with 100 workers at a factory that loses 20 per cent of its work force each year, only 33 of the original group will still be working at the factory at the end of five years.

A *cross-sectional study* combines aspects of both case-control and cohort studies. A household survey of injuries in a community is an example of a cross-sectional study. Individuals are included simply because they are available at the time of the study. Cross-sectional studies are the simplest and least expensive type of study. They are suitable for descriptive and exploratory purposes. Because multiple outcomes and multiple exposures can be studied simultaneously, cross-sectional studies can generate hypotheses that can be tested in more rigorously designed efforts.

CONDUCTING CROSS-SECTIONAL SURVEYS

A cross-sectional survey is often the first step in any community injury control effort. Surveys which are simply 'fishing expeditions', efforts to collect as much data as possible in the hope that something important will emerge, are usually rewarded with inconclusiveness and frustration. Elements that must be specified at the outset are:

- the nature of the injuries to be studied: intentional, occupational, etc.
- the level of severity of injuries: medically-treated, hospitalized, deaths.
- the target population: ages, geographic location, occupations.

Questionnaires and record-abstract forms are the most common survey instruments. Other approaches include direct observations, physical examinations, laboratory tests, and environmental measurements. For example, to study injuries among children working in small manufacturing establishments, a researcher can:

- review medial records of children treated for injuries,
- visit factories and ask the child workers if they have had an occupational injury,
- observe whether there are dangerous machines or other obvious hazards in the workplace,
- examine the workers for scars, burns, missing fingers, or other signs of injury,
- perform blood tests for lead exposure, and
- measure noise levels or asbestos fibers in the air at the factories.

Choosing which instrument or combination of instruments will be most appropriate depends on the objectives of the survey and the resources available. Decisions about appropriate sample size and sampling frameworks can be complicated. A statistician should be consulted early in the planning stage, not after the survey has been completed.

Designing a Survey Form

Data recording forms are often too lengthy and too complicated. Their designers hope to guarantee that nothing is left out that might be useful for future analysis. Extensive and complicated protocols are feasible when special injury investigating teams are established for in-depth, on-site studies of road traffic injuries, for example, certain team members are specially trained for long-term data collection. However, when long and complicated forms are distributed to persons such as doctors or police officers whose primary job is not data collection, the effort is frequently counterproductive:

–   The data may be inaccurate, incomplete, or both because the persons collecting the data may not have any real interest in epidemiological issues. Doctors are mainly interested in treating patients, not completing charts or forms. Police at the site of a motor vehicle crash are more interested in clearing the road for traffic and recording information for legal purposes. Doctors in emergency wards of hospitals may not be willing to spend more than a minute in recording epidemiologic details; police officer might be willing to spend up to five minutes.

–   The data may be unreliable because the persons collecting it may not be equipped to record it accurately. For example, traffic police without breathalyzers cannot reliably accurately identify intoxicated drivers; primary health care workers usually will be unable to diagnose internal injuries.

–   Extensive data forms make data collection and analysis much more expensive.

–   Much of the data never get used because it does not have any policy implications for instituting countermeasures.

To simplify data collection, specify the few critical issues which need to be addressed. A study on preventable causes of burns, for example, does not need to include information on how much colloid solution was used to treat each victim. Also, make the mechanics for completing the form as simple as possible. Provide checkoffs for the most common responses to a question or variable. Designate a section for the recorder to write in comments and descriptions, both to collect important details about the circumstances of injury and to reduce the number of items on the form. An uncomplicated form to record injury information in a rural village is shown in Table 3.4.

Table 3.4
Sample Village Injury Recording Form

Village Name _____

Name of Person Completing Form _____

Victim's Age _____ Sex _____ Date Injured _____ Time _____

Nature of Injury (e.g., fracture, cut) _____

Body Part Injured _____

Description of How Injury Happened _____

_____

_____

External Cause of Injury:

A. Motor Vehicle:

    Type: Motorcycle _____ Car _____ Bus ___ Other (state) _____

    Victim: Driver _____ Passenger _____ Pedestrian _____

    Bicyclist _____ Others (state) _____

B. Burn: Open Flame _____ Hot Liquid _____ Others (state) _____

C. Drowning _____

D. Poisoning (state substance) _____

E. Fall: Same Level _____ From Height _____

F. Others (state) _____

Outcome: Minor, Treated at Home _____

    Treated by Health Worker, Sent Home _____

    Sent to Hospital for Treatment, Released _____

    Admitted to Hospital _____

    Died Within 7 Days of Injury _____

Pilot Study

Even the most experienced researchers cannot predict every problem that may arise during data collection. A pilot study allows difficulties to surface before the large-scale survey is undertaken. Is there confusion about the meaning of certain questions? Are there overlapping categories for certain responses? How long does it actually take for an interviewer to drive to a residence, locate the 'head-of-household', and complete the interview? Where is a blood sample supposed to be stored if the laboratory is closed? These and other issues can be recognized by 'piloting' the survey on a small scale. Changes can then be made in the protocols, routines, and schedules so that the formal survey can proceed smoothly.

Several publications provide more in-depth discussions of important survey issues such as formulating questionnaires, selecting and training data collectors, and preparing the community for a survey.[2–4]

EVALUATION RESEARCH

There are at least three reasons why evaluating an intervention such as an educational campaign, a new law or an environmental change is important. First, if a programme is having a major impact this should be documented so the programme can be expanded and extended to other communities. If the intervention is having no impact or is actually having detrimental effects, this should be revealed so that scarce resources can be directed to more effective approaches. Second, the existence of most programmes depends on continued funding and interest. Programmes which lack evidence to support their claims of effectiveness are likely to lose their funding in times of economic cutbacks. Third, programmes involve commitments from parents, physicians, police, or project staff. Demonstrating that their time and energy are making a difference can guarantee continued support.

Planning an Evaluation

Evaluations require time and resources. Before embarking on any evaluation, the programme staff should have answers to the following questions:[5]

What are the specific goals and main objectives of the programme?

The design of any evaluation needs to be based on the programme's objectives. For example, if a programme seeks to reduce injuries from tractor rollovers on farms, different data needs to be collected than if the programme aims at reducing injuries from all types of machinery.[6]

What is the purpose of the evaluation?

Programme planners and staff need to agree on both the purpose of the evaluation and what will be done with the evaluation results. Is the evaluation intended to improve the operation of the programme? To demonstrate if the programme was effective or not? To determine if the expense justified the results? For whom is the evaluation intended—Funding agencies? Programme managers? The community? Answers to these questions will determine if the evaluation should be done by programme staff (internal evaluation) or outsiders (external evaluation); whether economic data will be collected; and how comprehensive the evaluation should be.

What resources—financial and human—are available for designing and conducting the evaluation?

Staff time is required to plan the evaluation, interview personnel and participants, collect data, code forms, analyse, and report the results. Costs are involved in retaining consultants, printing and mailing forms, holding meetings, and using computers. A simple evaluation may involve a single staff member telephoning a number of participants; a complicated one might involve thousands of rupees for analysis of costs and health outcomes.

Approaches to Evaluation

Structure, process, outcome and cost are aspects of any programme that can be evaluated. 'Structure' refers to the working components, the quantity and quality of facilities, equipment and personnel. For example, how many protective devices are available to workers in a factory injury prevention programme? What are the qualifications of the prevention staff? Are the facilities for emergency treatment of injured workers adequate?

'Process' evaluation looks at the programme's organization and activities. How many individuals received training in a first aid course? What characterized the individuals who participated and those who did not? During what hours were public service announcements broadcast on television? How many drunk-driving arrests were made during an enforcement campaign? What problems (insufficient funds, disagreements among key individuals, lack of manpower or other resources) interfered with implementation and how were they solved? Was there effective intersectoral coordination?

The *effects* or *outcomes* of injury prevention programmes can be measured as changes in knowledge, attitudes, behaviours, environment and, most importantly, rates of deaths and injuries. Has a pedestrian safety programme actually reduced the rate of pedestrian injuries in the previous year? Did the motorcyclists death rate fall after a mandatory helmet law was passed? Did the incidence of dog bites decline after an animal control programme began in a community?

Analysis of *costs* is essential because the funds available for any activity are not infinite. Also, agencies and individuals who provide financial support to programmes want assurances that their money is being well spent. One way to decide if the expense of a programme is reasonable is to estimate the benefits of the programme and compare them to costs. Another approach is to compare the programme costs with the costs of other programmes providing similar service or having similar goals (See 'Economic costs of injuries' in Chapter Two).

Comparison Data

Nowhere is comparison data more important than in evaluation research. It is very tempting to initiate a programme, wait a few months or a year and then report how well the target group is doing. It is essential to have comparison data, however, to be certain that changes are actually due to the intervention, and not to other unrelated factors. One approach is to use comparison data from the past (historical control).

The Ministry of Labour in a country launched a campaign in 1986 to reduce industrial injuries. The incidence of workmen's compensation claims in 1987 was 500 per 10,000 workers. An historical comparison was made using data from 1977, when the claims incidence was 600 per 10,000 workers. The Ministry declared that its campaign was a success.

Of course, there are many other possible reasons why the rate of workmen's compensation claims may have decreased in the 10-year period 1977 to 1987: enforcement of the compensation law may have changed; new, safer industries may have replaced older, more dangerous ones; or the eligibility requirements for compensation may have been re-written.

A different approach is to use a simultaneous comparison group:

An educational programme to prevent home injuries to children is to be evaluated in a private medical practice. The goal of the programme is to reduce the number of household hazards to children by making parents more aware of dangerous situations and substances. To evaluate the programme, parents bringing their children to the pediatrician for immunizations are randomized to either receive the education programme or not. One month later, a research assistant makes a surprise visit to the homes of all the families. The average number of hazards discovered in the homes of the families receiving the educational programme is compared to the average in the homes of the comparison families.

The problem with measuring the outcome only after the intervention is that the researcher cannot be certain (even with randomization) that the homes had the same number of hazards before the study began. The best evaluation design would be to have data on both the programme population *and* a comparison population before and after the programme is put into effect.

A health department wants to know if it should begin child car seat loaner programmes for low-income families. A survey is done in which trained observers at four health clinics note the proportion of infants in cars who are secured in safety seats. Two clinics are then randomly chosen to begin loaner programmes. One year later, the observers find that the proportion of infants in seats has risen from 10 per cent to 40 per cent at the 'loaner' clinics; at the other two clinics without the programme, the proportion has gone from 10 per cent to 12 per cent. The programme is deemed a success and instituted at all health department clinics.

An elegant 'real-world' example of the importance of a comparison
groups in evaluation research concerns firearm-related injuries in
Canada and the US:

> There are more than 32,000 firearm deaths each year in the United
> States, nearly the same as the number of deaths from breast cancer
> and diabetes.[7] About 12,000 of these deaths are homicides (murders),
> three-fourths of which involve handguns.[8] Steadily rising rates of
> firearm-related homicides and suicides in the US, associated with
> skyrocketing sales of new firearms (Figure 3.1), has prompted calls
> for stricter regulations on the purchase and possession of firearms.[7]
> Opponents of handgun regulations argue that these laws are not ef-
> fective, that they will not keep guns from criminals, but will restrict
> their use by law-abiding citizens for self-defense.
>
> To assess the impact of handgun regulations, street crimes and
> homicides were studied in Seattle, Washington (a city in the northwest
> corner of the United States) and Vancouver, British Columbia (a city
> in Canada, just 233 km north of Seattle) from 1980 through 1986.[8]
> Similar to Seattle in many ways (education levels, climate, geography,
> history, income, unemployment rates), Vancouver has much more
> restrictive handgun regulations. In Seattle, handguns may be legally

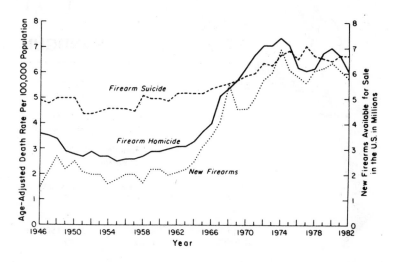

Figure 3.1: Increases in firearm-related homicides and suicides have paral-
leled the increased availability of firearms in the United States. Wintemute,
G. J., Firearms as a cause of death in the United States. Journal of Trauma,
Volume 27, Number 5, pp. 532–5, copyright by Williams and Wilkins, 1987.

purchased for self-defense, a permit can be obtained to carry a handgun as a concealed weapon, and there are minimal restrictions on the recreational use of handguns. In Vancouver, self-defence is not a valid or legal reason to purchase a handgun, concealed weapons are not permitted, and strict regulations exist on the transport and recreational use of handguns (e.g., for target shooting or collecting).

The rate of assaults involving firearms was seven times higher in Seattle than in Vancouver. The risk of being murdered with a handgun in Seattle was 4.8 times higher than Vancouver. Both cities had similar rates of burglary, robbery, assaults not involving firearms, and homicide by other means than guns.

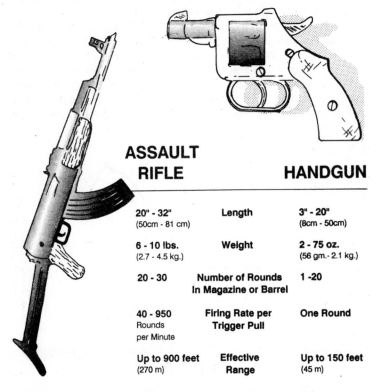

ASSAULT RIFLE		HANDGUN
20" - 32" (50cm - 81 cm)	**Length**	3" - 20" (8cm - 50cm)
6 - 10 lbs. (2.7 - 4.5 kg.)	**Weight**	2 - 75 oz. (56 gm.- 2.1 kg.)
20 - 30	**Number of Rounds in Magazine or Barrel**	1 -20
40 - 950 Rounds per Minute	**Firing Rate per Trigger Pull**	One Round
Up to 900 feet (270 m)	**Effective Range**	Up to 150 feet (45 m)

Figure 3.2: Handguns are the most common type of firearm involved in homicides and suicides in the United States. Assault rifles and their modifications are popular among dealers of illegal drugs (such as heroin and cocaine).

Sound evaluation research, such as the Seattle/Vancouver study, and recent public outrage about epidemics of murder (many drug-related) involving military style weapons called assault rifles, may convince national and state legislators to pass stricter laws regulating firearms (Figure 3.2).

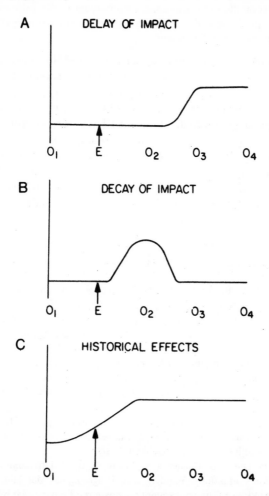

Figure 3.3: The timing of observations (O) and experimental interventions (E) can greatly alter the conclusions of an evaluation. From Green, L. W., Evaluation and measurement: Some dilemmas for health education. *Am J Public Health* 1977, **67**:155–8. Copyright, *American Journal of Public Health*.

Timing of Evaluations

The Minister of Child Health for a country becomes alarmed at the high rate of drownings among children in rural areas. She decides that a massive public education campaign is needed. Sound trucks urge children to stay away from canals and open wells. Messages are broadcast on the radio and appear on billboards. After the campaign has been implemented, the Director orders another survey of drownings, the rate has not changed.

Was the drowning prevention campaign a failure? Not necessarily the follow-up survey may have occurred either too soon or too late to see an impact (Figure 3.3).[9] The survey may have been performed before most of the people had a chance to hear or view the messages (delay of impact). Alternatively, it may have been conducted long after the messages had an effect (decay of impact).

These two examples demonstrate the value of serial observations (also called time series analysis) for evaluation research. Although 'before and after' observations are useful, repeated measurements over time offer additional insights into important trends.

REFERENCES

1. Rainey, D. Y., Runyan, C. W. 1992. Newspapers: A source of injury surveillance? *American Journal of Public Health* 82: 745–6.
2. Lutz, W. 1981. *Planning and Organising a Health Survey: A Guide for Health Workers.* International Epidemiological Association, Geneva. Division of Health Statistics, WHO, 1211 Geneva 27, Switzerland.
3. The National Committee for Injury Prevention and Control: 1989. *Injury Prevention: Meeting the Challenge.* Published by Oxford University Press as a supplement to the American Journal of Preventive Medicine, Volume 5, Number 3.
4. Training manual on research and action methodologies and techniques concerning the health of working children. Maternal and Child Health, World Health Organization, Geneva, 1987.
5. Lantz, P., Lee, B. C., Gallagher, S., Young, N. B. 1993. Evaluation Guidebook for Community Youth Safety Programmes, Marshfield Clinic, Marshfield, Rural Injury Prevention Resource Center, 1000 North Oak Avenue, Marshfield, WI 54449–5790, USA.
6. Surgeon General's Conference on Agricultural Safety and Health, 1991. *Morbidity and Mortality Weekly Report* 1992; 41 (1): 5, 11–12.

7. Wintemute, G. J. 1987. Firearms as a cause of death in the United States, 1920–82. *The Journal of Trauma* **27**: 532–6.
8. Sloan, J. H., Kellermann, A. L., Reay, D. T. et al. 1988. Handgun regulations, crime, assaults, and homicide: A tale of two cities. *New England Journal of Medicine* **319**: 1256.
9. Greene, L. W. 1977. Evaluation and measurement: Some dilemmas for health education. *American Journal of Public Health* **67**: 155–8.

FURTHER READINGS

1. Health Research Methodology: A Guide for Training in Research Methods. WHO Regional Office for the Western Pacific, Manila, 1992.
2. Pietrzak, J., Ramler, M., Renner, T., Ford, L., Gilbert, N. 1990. *Practical Programme Evaluation: Examples from Child Abuse Prevention*, Sage Publications, Newbury Park.
3. Lwanga, S. K., Tye, C. Y. 1986. Teaching Health Statistics, WHO, Geneva.
4. Weiss, C. H. 1972. *Evaluation Research*, Prentice Hall, New Jersey.

4

The Human Body's Response to Transfers of Energy

Advances in the prevention of injuries and reduction in their severity often come from an understanding of the body's response to injury-producing energies. The three major sections of this chapter illustrate how a scientific understanding of injury mechanisms contributes to injury control. Biomechanical principles, for example, underlay injuries related to mechanical (kinetic) energy. Anatomic and physiologic information can help prevent injuries from all forms of energy: thermal, mechanical, chemical, radiation, and electrical. An appreciation of the physiologic effects of alcohol, other drugs, and medical conditions helps explain their role in motor vehicle crashes.

Obviously, each of these sections are enormous topics in their own right. The purpose of the brief discussions which follow is to highlight the role of basic and applied sciences in injury control.

BIOMECHANICS AND INJURY CONTROL

Biomechanics is an interdisciplinary field which combines physics, mechanical engineering, and life sciences to understand the relationship of physical forces to the functioning of the human body. Basic researchers in biomechanics study such phenomenon as the mechanics of muscle function and respiration. Applied researchers help design equipment for orthopaedic rehabilitation, surgical implants, and sports safety.

An important concept of biomechanics is that of human tolerance, there are quantifiable limits to the human's ability to withstand physical forces without harm. If these limits are exceeded, reversible or irreversible injury will occur. Human tolerance limits vary with different types of physical input such as impact, acceleration, vibration, compression, stretch, bending and twisting of tissues and body segments. Much of biomechanics research, both basic and applied investigates what kind and severity of injuries are caused by what magnitude and kind of physical inputs. This information can then be used to design both protective devices and environments.

Biomechanics is valuable in studying all three phases of injury: pre-event, event and post-event (see Chapter Six). In the pre-event phase, biomechanics often overlaps with ergonomics in designing products and environments that improve working postures and movements, and minimize the likelihood of injury during work or leisure. In the event phase, the role of biomechanics is to provide human tolerance data to prevent injuries or reduce their severity in the event of a crash or fall, or as a result of forces released in the course of occupational or sports activities. For example, biomechanical knowledge has been used to design:

- Laminated windshields, padded dashboards and knee bolsters, collapsible steering columns, air bags and seat belts in cars,
- Child car safety seats and safety helmets,
- Vibration reduction seats in tractors and trucks,
- Safer bindings in skis and safer running shoes,
- Safety standards for children's toys and furniture and play grounds,
- Standards for construction sites and codes for lifting loads safely.

During the post-event phase, biomechanical research has led to the design of better fixators, pins, nails and braces for treating fractures, to a better understanding of the mechanisms of bed sores and improved methods of surgical and non-surgical treatment, and to a scientific approach to the design of individual prosthetics, orthotics, and physiotherapy regimens during injury rehabilitation.

Methods of Biomechanics Research

A great deal of useful information about mechanical forces and injuries can be obtained by studying real life injury events. An example is Hugh DeHaven's pioneering work on falls from heights.[1] DeHaven measured the 'drop height' of humans in non-fatal falls from high buildings. By correlating the drop height, the properties of the object struck, and the indentation, he was able to show that the human body can survive relatively high decelerations when the resulting forces are widely distributed over the surface of the body. Also in the early 1940's, Sir Hugh Cairns studied fatalities and head injuries among army dispatch riders.[2, 3] He found that many of the head injuries occurred at the sides of the head. Riders who wore helmets had less severe injuries. Such studies provided the basis for modern day motorcycle helmets which provide protection for the entire head and face.

However, more detailed biomechanical data is necessary to design a protective helmet for football players or a bullet-proof vest for police officers or a collapsible steering wheel that does not impale a driver's chest in the event of a collision. Studies of real-life injuries usually cannot provide sufficient quantitative data about the injury producing forces. A variety of experimental methods are, therefore, used to assess biomechanical forces and human tolerance limits.

Use of artificial systems

Anthropomorphic (human-like) dummies are widely used in experiments on crash protection. Helmets are tested using an artificial head fitted with accelerometers. Seat belt studies use a dummy with an artificial thorax whose deflection characteristics simulate those of the human body. Injuries to other body parts such as the face can be studied with customized monitoring devices like the 'load-sensing face' (LSF):

> Sled tests were carried out with a LSF-equipped dummy to study the pressure time histories for various impact conditions. Impact locations and severity as well as duration and time sequence of the impact were evaluated. The LSF showed a good ability to distinguish between changes in impact conditions, for example for a different seating position. . . Passenger pressure results were of a much lower magnitude than that for the driver.[4]

Of course, the extent to which a particular dummy simulates its human counterpart is of enormous importance (and often a point of considerable debate). A great advantage of these 'artificial humans' is that they can be reproduced in quantity and fully standardized, making comparison studies possible.[5, 6]

Use of volunteers

One of the first and classic studies involving the use of a human volunteer in biomechanical research was conducted by Colonel John Stapp. Stapp subjected himself to high accelerations in a rocket sled.[7] He kept increasing the acceleration of the sled until he suffered retinal hemorrhage and unconsciousness. His studies proved conclusively that many car crashes are survivable if the human body can be prevented from hitting hard structures inside the car. These principles led to the design of life-saving lap and shoulder belts and air bags for cars. Human volunteers have also participated in research to determine the range of neck movement of human beings,[8] the compression properties of the chest,[9] low back lifting capabilities,[10] forces in gymnastic activities,[11] and forces on the foot during running.[12] A great deal of work has also been done to improve artificial limbs using instrumented human volunteers.[13, 14]

The advantage of using volunteers is that human physiology and anatomy can be studied under real life conditions while physical parameters are simultaneously measured. The drawbacks are that there are clear limitations on the kind of measuring devices that can be used (e.g., they must not themselves injure the volunteer or increase the risk of an injury). Also, the forces to which volunteers can be subjected have to be kept much below injury levels (tolerance thresholds are approached from the bottom up). However, such studies can give very valuable data that lead to formal safety policies and regulations:

> To determine the strength needed to hold an infant during an automobile crash, an adult subject was seated on an automobile bench which was rigidly fixed (Figure 4.1). A lap-and-shoulder belt was locked in position. The adult held an infant dummy weighing 7.9 kg with anthropometric dimensions of a 6-month old infant. In dynamic tests, a cable was pulled by a piston to simulate crash forces. Force transducers (load cells) were attached to the lap belt, shoulder belt, and the cable; a displacement transducer was attached to the cable to measure cable position. Results clearly demonstrated that an infant in a 50 km/hr crash would almost certainly strike the dash or windshield of the car, even when held tightly by a restrained adult.[15]

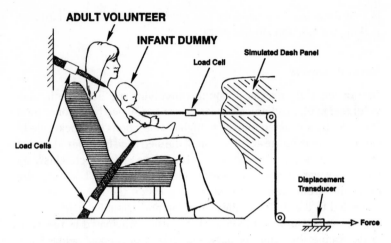

ADULT VOLUNTEER

INFANT DUMMY

Load Cell

Simulated Dash Panel

Load Cells

Displacement
Transducer

Force

Figure 4.1: A biomechanics experiment in which an infant
dummy is pulled from the lap of a restraining adult. Load
cells measure the forces involved. From *Human Factors*,
Volume 21, Number 6, December 1979; Copyright 1979 by The
Human Factors Society, Inc., and reproduced by permission.

Use of human cadavers

Research involving human cadavers makes it possible to fill in gaps
in knowledge obtained from animal experiments, reconstruction of
'real-life' crashes, and human volunteer studies. Since cadavers have
almost the same dimensions and geometry as living human beings,
and because bone properties do not change appreciably after death,
data from cadaver research can be used to validate computer models
and to design test dummies. Research with cadavers has other ad-
vantages: a wide variety of measuring devices can be used, and
testing can be done to the point of destruction (which is especially
important in the study of fractures or internal injuries).

An example of the value of postmortem human subjects (cadavers)
is their use in studying motor vehicle crashes. Highway crashes in
which people were killed or injured can be simulated in the laboratory using cadavers and mechanical sleds accelerated to varying
velocities. Impact forces can be measured by attaching accelerometers to the cadavers. The injuries sustained in the laboratory are
then compared to those which occurred in the 'real-life' crashes. The

different sets of data then give an indication of what kind of physical damage can be expected with a given range of forces, accelerations, sitting positions, and so on.[16, 17]

There are several disadvantages to injury research using cadavers. Observation of secondary effects such as development of cerebral edema after a skull fracture is often impossible. Distortions are introduced because post-mortem anatomy differs from living structures (e.g., muscle tone is absent). Large biological variations among cadavers means that considerable caution must be exercised in applying the research results. Cadaver research obviously can be done only in the relatively few countries that have legislation governing the donation of human bodies to science.

Animal experiments

Experiments with animals allow researchers to study physiologic processes and the responses of living tissues to biomechanical forces. Many of the early studies on tolerance to impact involved research with animals. Animals are used less often for injury research today. Knowing that a small monkey can withstand a peak acceleration of 2000g is of limited applicability to humans, especially when there is now available a great deal of human specific tolerance data. Also, growing public support for the protection of animals in laboratories places increasing constraints on experiments. Only when other types of research cannot produce the data essential for protecting humans should animal studies be considered.

Computer models

Computers have been used, for example, to study the kinetics of motor vehicle/pedestrian collisions. Computer simulations can model how different parts of the anatomy will be impacted when a person is struck by a vehicle. The model can be changed for persons of different ages, heights, and weights and for different vehicles at varying speeds. The value of the computer simulation depends largely on the accuracy of the designer's data about the real-life situation. It is just as easy to run an unrealistic model as an accurate one. The use of computer models therefore depends on continuous matching of results against data from the real world.

Many of today's computer crash/injury models have taken a long time (almost twenty years) to develop and are very complex.[18-21] They are being used to refine biomechanical experiments and to improve the designs of vehicles and protective devices. Computers are especially valuable in sensitivity analyses, predicting injury outcomes under a variety of crash conditions. For example, computer modelling revealed that in most crash situations, crash forces on both the neck and head decrease when a motorcycle rider is wearing a helmet.[22]

What follows are examples of how biomechanical research has already led to dramatic reductions in injuries.

Biomechanics and Motor Vehicle Occupant Injuries

In the United States, motor vehicle crashes cause two thirds of all hospitalized injuries involving the liver, spleen and chest organs (heart or lung); more than half of all spinal cord injuries; and nearly half of all head injuries, pelvic fractures and severe facial injuries (Table 4.1).[23] As in all injuries, the most important factors in determining the severity of injuries in a frontal car crash relate to the host,

Table 4.1
Hospitalized Injuries Caused by Motor Vehicle Crashes*

Site of Injury	Per cent Due to M.V. Crashes
Heart or lung	65
Liver	65
Spleen	58
Kidney	43
Pneumo-/hemo-thorax	40
Intestine	38
Distal femur fracture	44
Pelvis fracture	40
Patella fracture	38
Head	39

Note: * Rhode Island Residents, 1979–1980. Adapted from Fife, reference 22.

On impact, the car begins to crush and slow down. The person inside continues to move forward at 35 mph.

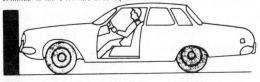

Within 1/10 of a second, the car comes to a stop, but the person keeps moving forward at 35 mph.

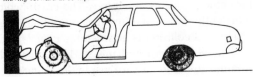

1/50 of a second after the car has stopped, the unbelted person slams into the dashboard or windshield. This is the human collision.

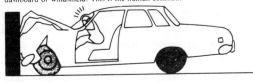

Only with *effective* seat belts will the person stop before his or her head or chest hits the steering wheel, dash, or windshield.

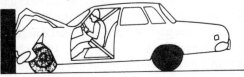

Figure 4.2: The sequence of events in a car crash, with and without use of a lap-shoulder seat belt. From Gillis, J. and Fierst, K., *The Car Book*, Harper and Row, New York, 1987, p. 26.

agent and environment: design features of the car and roadside, the speed of the vehicle (or vehicles) at the time of the crash, and whether the occupants are restrained by protective devices. Car features that can increase occupant injuries are protruding knobs on the dashboard, windshields that shatter into tiny fragments, rigid steering wheels that can impale drivers, seat backs without head supports, and exterior bodies made from plastic or inexpensive steel.[24] Rigid and sharp objects (such as hood ornaments or metal bumper guards) attached to the front of motor vehicles can inflict severe injuries on pedestrians and two-wheeler riders. Examples of roadside hazards are concrete signs and lamp-posts, ditches, sturdy trees, and sharp-edged barriers that can penetrate cars (Photo 5.1).

There has been extensive research on the biomechanics of motor vehicle occupant injuries.[25-27] Consider the situation where a driver is not wearing a seat belt, swerves to avoid an animal on the highway, and the motor vehicle crashes into a tree. The crash, which occurs in less than one-tenth of a second involves more than one collision (Figure 4.2).[28] The first collision is between the *vehicle* and the tree. As the front end of the car is crushed, the car decelerates. The driver, however, continues to move forward inside the vehicle at the car's initial speed. The *second* collision—the *human collision*—occurs a fraction of a second after the first, when the driver strikes the interior of the car at the windshield, dashboard, and steering wheel. The collision of internal organs against each other, brain against skull, spleen against rib cage, can be considered a third collision.

The impact energy increases in proportion to the square of the car's velocity.[29] Impact forces are roughly proportional to the deceleration of the body during impact. Impact forces can be twice as great when a car hits a barrier at 110 km/hr hour compared to 80 km/hr. As a car's impact speed rises above 30 kmph the likelihood of death in a frontal crash increases sharply; at 65 kmph it is ten times greater and at 80 kmph it is *twenty* times greater.[30]

Crash force on an unrestrained adult occupant can be over 60,000 Newtons (9.81 Newtons is the force exerted by 1 kg acting under the influence of gravity). Yet, these forces on the body can be reduced by distributing them over time (reducing the amount of deceleration) or by distributing them over a wider area of the body. Seat belts perform both functions and can actually prevent the second collision.[31] For children too small to use seat belts, special restraint devices are needed (Figure 4.3).[32-34] Adults cannot protect children from injury in a crash by holding them tightly on their laps (see experimental methods above). Also, if the adult is not wearing a seat belt during a crash, the child can be crushed between the adult and the car's interior.

An air cushion system is also very effective in protecting occupants from injury as a result of frontal impacts.[35-38] Unlike manual

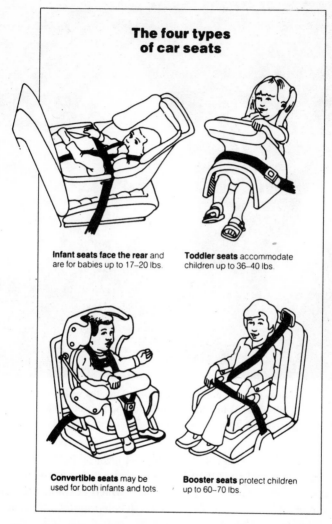

**The four types
of car seats**

Infant seats face the rear and are for babies up to 17–20 lbs.

Toddler seats accommodate children up to 36–40 lbs.

Convertible seats may be used for both infants and tots.

Booster seats protect children up to 60–70 lbs.

Figure 4.3: Car safety devices for children require an informed public to purchase the appropriate type and use it correctly. From Forster, J. H., Car safety seats. Contemporary Pediatrics, November 1984, pp. 59–72, copyright Medical Economics.

seat belts that require occupants to buckle them up before driving, air cushions protect automatically (Photo 4.1). When a frontal crash

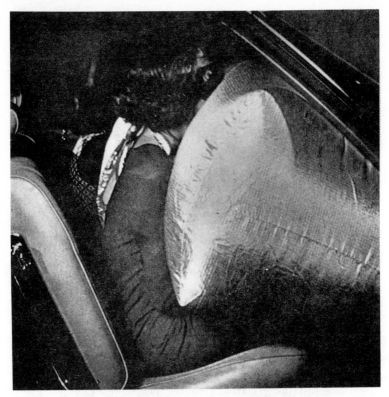

Photo 4.1: An air cushion (air bag) inflates with inert nitrogen gas in a fraction of a second to protect car occupants from frontal injuries. (Courtesy of NHTSA.)

occurs, electrical or mechanical sensors trigger an inflator filled with inert gas. The air bag is then inflated in a fraction of a second. The occupants move forward into the bags, which cushion them from the forces of impact. The air cushions deflate rapidly after reaching their maximum inflation.

About 90 per cent of the 1994 model cars in the United States have air bags, either driver side only or 'dual systems' protecting both drivers and front-seat passengers. Dozens of models being sold in Europe and Japan are also equipped with air bags. In frontal crashes involving large cars, there is a 35 per cent reduction in driver deaths when the vehicles have air bags.[35]

Biomechanics and Motorcyclist Head Injuries

Per unit of travel, motorcyclists are five to twenty-times more likely to be killed than the occupants of other vehicles.[39, 40] Head injuries are the most common cause of death while the extremities are more often involved in non-lethal injuries.[41]

There are three general categories of head injury: fractures, other focal injuries, and diffuse brain injuries (Table 4.2).[42] It is damage to the vascular and neural elements of the brain, not fractures of the cranial vault alone, that lead to neurologic disability and death.

Table 4.2[*]
Types of Head Injuries

Skull Fractures:
Linear
Depressed
Basilar
Focal Injuries:
Hematomas: epidural, subdural, intracerebral
Contusions: coup, contracoup, intermediate
Diffuse Brain Injuries:
Concussion
Diffuse axonal injury

Note: [*] Adapted from Gennarelli, reference 42.

Head injuries can be caused by direct impacts (such as a motorcyclist falling onto a pavement) or by forces generated by sudden acceleration or deceleration (e.g., whiplash injuries). *Contact injuries* involve a blow to the head; head motion is not necessary to produce these injuries. They include skull fractures, extradural and intracerebral hematomas, and brain contusions. *Acceleration injuries* require head motion; a direct blow to the head is not necessary. Brain contusions, concussion syndromes, subdural hematomas, and diffuse axonal injuries can all be caused by acceleration/deceleration forces. Most clinical situations involve both head contact and head motion.[43]

The effectiveness of safety helmets in preventing serious head injury has been confirmed repeatedly through both biomechanical and real-world studies.[44] One such study involved crashes where the pavement was the only surface against which the motorcyclist struck his head. Riders with helmets suffered only minor injuries at a rate of 23 per 1000 crashes. Riders without helmets had 65 brain injuries per 1,000 crashes, many of them serious or critical.[45] Opponents of helmet laws claim that helmets increase the risk of spinal cord injuries to the neck. The claim is without foundation, an in-depth study of 846 non-fatal motorcycle crashes found not a single spinal cord injury.[45] As noted above, a computer modelling study of head impacts showed that helmets actually reduce neck forces under most situations.[22]

Biomechanics research has produced improvements in windshields, dashboards, steering columns, and restraint systems in cars.[46] These improvements have saved tens of thousands of lives and prevented hundreds of thousands of injuries to vehicle occupants.[47] Among the priorities for biomechanical research in injury prevention are the design of vehicles that can protect occupants in high-speed crashes;[48, 49] motorcycle helmets that are crash-effective, inexpensive, and comfortable to wear in hot climates; and more forgiving fronts of vehicles (such as buses and trucks) to minimize injuries to pedestrians and two-wheeler riders (see Chapter Six).

ANATOMY AND PHYSIOLOGY OF INJURIES

Scald Burns

Nature of the problem

Scald burns are thermal injuries caused by hot liquids. In the Netherlands, a country of 14.5 million people, some 45,000 people visit a hospital for the treatment of scalds each year;[50] In the United States, between 2,400 and 4,500 people are hospitalized with these burns.[51] The most common liquids causing burns are hot water, coffee, and tea. Toddlers and pre-school children are injured most frequently. The burns are often severe and extend over large portions of the body, as when a child unintentionally pulls a pot of boiling water on himself or herself. Scald burns also occur as child abuse, when a parent intentionally places a youngster in very hot water to frighten or punish the child. In many countries, scald burns are the most common reason for children to be hospitalized with burns.

Anatomic and physiologic considerations

For any individual, the severity of a scald burn depends on the temperature of the liquid and the length of time it is in contact with the skin. As shown in Figure 4.4, adult skin will suffer a full-thickness burn after two seconds of exposure to water at 65° C (150° F); a full minute is required when the water temperature is (127° F).[51]

The age and sex of the victim is also important. Infants and children

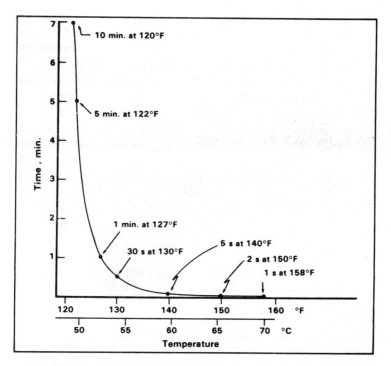

Figure 4.4: The duration of exposure needed to cause a third-degree burn in adult skin varies with the temperature of the water. Guzzetta, P. C. and Randolph, J., Burns in Children: 1982. Pediatrics in Review, Volume 4, No. 9, March, 1983, pp. 271–8. Copyright 1983, American Academy of Pediatrics. Reproduced with permission.

have a much thinner dermis than adults, making full thickness burns more likely at lower temperatures and shorter time exposures. Females have fewer hair follicles than males, reducing the number of deep-dermal cells available for primary healing of a severe burn. A child with a mental or physical handicap is at particular risk of scald injury. Impaired temperature sensation or motor disabilities can prolong the time a child is exposed to excessively hot water. Also, thinner skin over paralytic extremities may burn more quickly.[52] Elderly persons with cerebrovascular problems, epilepsy, arthritis, and cataracts are also at risk for scald burns, particularly while carrying containers with hot liquids at home.[50]

Implications for prevention

- In homes with hot-water heaters, the temperature of tap water can be over 75.5° C (168° F).[53] By lowering the thermostat setting, the water temperatures could be reduced to a safer 49° C (120° F) or less. This will reduce the likelihood of tap water scald burns from all causes, intentional and unintentional.
- When a person's clothing becomes soaked with hot liquid, contact with the skin is prolonged, leading to more severe burns. Pouring cold water on the person—or removing the clothing as quickly as possible, if cold water is not immediately available—will reduce the severity of the burn.[54]
- Groups at highest risk of scald burns are pre-school children, children with physical and mental handicaps, and elderly adults with conditions that affect their alertness, vision, or mobility.

Asphyxia from Small Parts

Nature of the problem

Putting things in the mouth is a developmentally normal way for infants and young children to explore their environment. However, many objects are small enough to occlude airways if aspirated. For example, nine children died by inhaling the tops of pens in the United Kingdom between 1970 and 1984. Even toys, pacifiers, and rattles have parts that can occlude the trachea. Partial airway occlusion can cause anoxia, atelectasis, pneumonia, and permanent lung damage.[55]

In the United States, more than 7,000 children under 10 years of age are treated in emergency rooms for injuries related to small parts. Of the incidents involving choking, 80 per cent are children under three years of age.[56] With over 1,500 toy manufacturers producing more than 150,000 different toys worldwide each year,[57] simple tests for excluding hazardous objects are necessary.

Anatomic and Physiologic considerations

The Consumer Safety Unit of the Department of Trade and Industry in the UK decided to investigate the pen-top problem. They commissioned the Royal Victoria Infirmary and the Department of Mechanical Engineering of the University of Newcastle-upon-Tyne, to carry out air-flow tests on tracheal models. The tests showed that pen tops with smooth, cylindrical surfaces did not allow sufficient air flow (four liters per minute) to sustain life until bronchoscopic removal was possible. A design that did allow sufficient flow is shown in Figure 4.5. This top has a pocket clip attached to the cap itself; the clip extends the full length of the cap, and when viewed end-on, there is a minimum of 5 mm^2 of space in cross-section beneath the clip.[58]

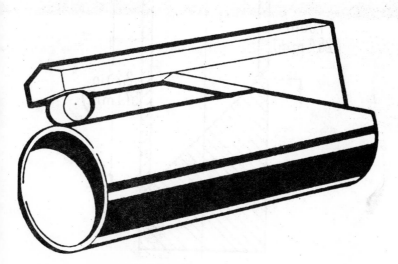

Figure 4.5: Recommended pen top to prevent aspiration deaths among children. From ECPSA Newsletter, Volume 2, No. 4, December, 1986, p. 6.

A review of death certificates and injury reports indicated that objects ranging in size from ³⁄₁₆ inch (0.5 cm) to 1¾ inches (4.4 cm) in greatest diameter can produce fatal obstruction of the air passages.

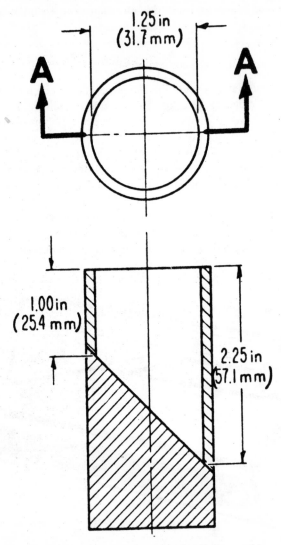

Figure 4.6: The dimensions of the truncated cylinder used to screen toys for dangerous small parts. Reproduced from the US Federal Register.

Small objects obviously can come in many different shapes, making a single design requirement impossible. Therefore, the US Consumer Product Safety Commission designed a 'small parts cylinder' whose truncated shape is similar to the lower portion of the pharynx. If an object in any orientation fits entirely within the cylinder, it fails the test. The cylinder screens long slender objects (such as pins) as well as bulkier objects, such as small balls (Figure 4.6). Objects that are larger than the cylinder are subjected to a 'use and abuse' procedure. Any pieces that become detached during the procedure are also tested in the cylinder. The regulations apply to all toys and other articles intended for use by children under 36 months of age.[55]

Implications for prevention

- Toys, furniture, and other products intended for children should be stringently evaluated for possible choking hazards. Both the presence of small parts and the object's sturdiness (resistance to being torn, hammered, or bitten into inhalable pieces) deserve attention.
- Pacifiers, intended to be placed in children's mouths should not be manufactured of parts that can separate. They should be made of a single piece of non-toxic material with wide flanges (at least 44 mm in diameter) and an easily-grasped handle.[59, 60]
- Foods such as nuts and vitamin tablets that require a grinding motion of the teeth to chew them adequately should be not be given to young children.
- Design modifications may reduce the risk of other aspiration hazards, such as certain foods and common household objects.[61]

Lead Poisoning

Nature of the problem

Lead is one of the best known, and most widespread, toxic substances in the environment.[62] Each year in the United States alone, over one million metric tons of lead are consumed by industry, with more than half being released into the environment. The Centers for

Disease Control describes childhood lead poisoning as 'one of the most common environmental diseases of children in the United States'.[63]

Lead poisoning can be acute or chronic, clinically obvious or asymptomatic. In severe lead poisoning (usually at blood lead levels over 100 µg/100 ml in adults) seizures, coma, and death can result. Earlier signs and symptoms in adults include colic, wrist or ankle extensor muscle weakness, irritability, decreased attention span, headache, hallucinations, and memory loss. Anemia and elevated blood urea nitrogen levels are often present. Chronic exposures result in anemia, neurologic damage, renal disease and reproductive impairment. Even the fetus is not immune; congenital lead poisoning has occurred from maternal exposures to lead at work, in pottery glazes, cosmetics, and home-brewed alcoholic beverages.[64]

A syndrome of 'subclinical' lead poisoning can occur in children at lead levels once thought to be harmless (less than 25 micrograms per decilitre). Blood, kidney and neurologic effects have been described. Children with elevated body lead burdens, but who have never shown any signs of *acute* lead toxicity, have impaired performance on tests of verbal and reading ability, memory, concentration, and motor skills.[65, 66] Behavioural problems have been documented among children with blood lead levels over 15 µg/dl.[67]

The major routes of human exposure are shown in Figure 4.7. In HICs, lead smelters, leaded gasoline, and house paint containing lead are the major sources of exposure. Occupational exposures to lead occur in hundreds of industries: the lead smelting and refining industries, manufacture of electrical components and leaded glass, scrap smelters, storage battery and lead chemical plants, welding, soldering, paint scraping, brass and bronze foundries, and printing among them.[68] Children of workers from industries that use lead are often contaminated from dust brought home on the workers' clothes, shoes, and skin.

Lead-based paint has been a major source of high-dose lead exposure and asymptomatic lead poisoning for children in the United States. Lead paint was commonly used in houses built before 1940. Some paints contained more than 50 per cent (500,000 ppm) lead. Many of these houses, now dilapidated with the paint peeling from the walls and ceilings, have low income families living in them. The infants and toddlers put the paint chips and other lead-contaminated items in their mouths. Although titanium dioxide has replaced white

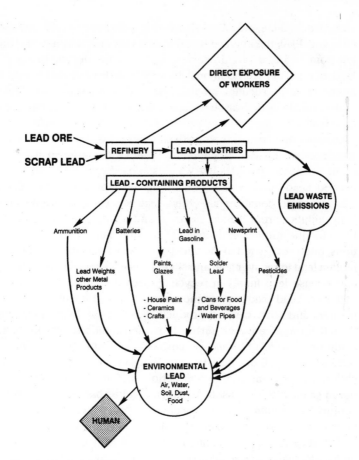

Figure 4.7: Lead exposures can occur from many different sources.

lead as a pigment, an estimated 27 million households in the US remain contaminated by lead paint.

Lead in the air is not only inhaled, it also falls onto soil, dust, and foliage where it can be ingested directly (especially by children whose hand-to-mouth activity is normal and extensive). Tetraethyl lead (TEL), added to gasoline to make engines run smoother, contributes about 90 per cent of the lead in the urban atmosphere. Soil and air lead levels are much higher around homes close to heavy motor vehicle traffic. An estimated 200,000 tons of lead were used in gasoline in the USA in the mid-1970's. Because most new cars run on *unleaded* gasoline, only about 2,000 tons were used in 1988. Between 1976 and 1980, the average blood lead levels in children in the USA fell from 14.6 to 9.2 μg/dl, corresponding to the decline in sales of leaded gasoline. An additional hazard from leaded gasoline is its abuse as an intoxicating inhalant. Reports of teenagers who deliberately inhale leaded gasoline vapors describe toxic encephalopathy and deaths.[69]

Lead in drinking occurs where lead pipes or copper pipes with lead solder have been used for plumbing. Where water is unusually acidic, as in Scotland, international water standards for lead can be exceeded. Lead can also enter food through lead solder used in canning.

Low-income countries also have lead smelters, severe airborne lead pollution from leaded gasoline, and lead paint. The LICs also have unique sources of toxic lead exposure. Small industrial operations, often conducted in the midst of crowded neighbourhoods, use molten lead to recover gold and silver from jewellers' waste materials and release lead fumes in recycling discarded automobile storage batteries. Lead oxide is common in glazes used for dishes, bowls, pitchers and other ceramic products. If not properly formulated or heated, the lead can leach out into foods and liquids, especially highly acidic ones. '*Kohl*' or '*surma*' is a cosmetic popular in Northern Africa, the Middle East, India, Pakistan, and Bangladesh. Women and young children apply it as an eye-liner (Photo 4.2). It often contains powdered galena, or lead disulfide, which can be absorbed through the conjunctiva. *Surma* has been documented as a source of both prenatal lead exposure and postnatal toxicity (including encephalopathy and death). Kuwait has banned the use of lead in *kohl*.[70] Folk remedies for various ailments (such as fever in among children from Thailand, stomach complaints in Mexican families) have caused outbreaks of lead poisoning as well. The Mexican folk remedy, called 'azarcon,' contains 86 per cent to 95 per cent lead tetroxide. Many severe poisonings occur when discarded automobile battery casings are burned for heat in the homes of poor families.[71]

Physiologic considerations

Lead has no known physiologic role in the body. It inhibits enzyme systems by forming metal complexes with various chemical (e.g., sulfhydryl) groups. Inhibition of delta-aminolevulinic acid dehydrate (delta-ALAD), an enzyme in the synthesis of haemoglobin, begins at

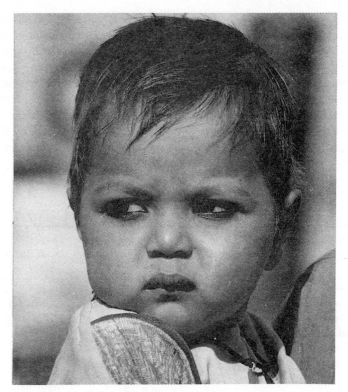

Photo 4.2: This child's dark eye shadow or *'surma'* might contain large amounts of lead. Absorbed through the conjunctiva, the lead can cause severe poisonings.

a blood lead level of 5 to 10 µg/dl; reduced haemoglobin levels can be seen at blood lead levels of 40 µg/dl and above.[63]

Kidney toxicity involves enzyme inhibition in the proximal tubules, including interference with vitamin D metabolism. Lead's ability to form stable chemical complexes is also the basis for the use of chelating agents (like penicillamine and calcium EDTA) in the treatment of lead poisoning.

Organic lead, such as TEL used in gasoline, is more lipid soluble than inorganic lead. It therefore can accumulate rapidly in the central nervous system and cause early and more severe neuropathy and encephalopathy.

Children absorb a larger proportion of lead from the gastrointestinal tract than adults (50 per cent vs 5–10 per cent). Once absorbed, lead is carried almost exclusively by erythrocytes. The majority of the absorbed lead is deposited in bone. Heavy deposition can impair bone growth, resulting in 'lead lines' on x-rays. During an acute illness, such as a bout of diarrhoea, lead can be rapidly mobilized from bone, resulting in signs of acute toxicity. Lead in teeth provides a measure of total body burden that can be assessed when children lose their primary dentition. Excretion of absorbed lead occurs mainly by the kidneys and to a lesser extent by the biliary tract. Adults retain little absorbed dietary lead; children retain 20–25 per cent.

Table 4.3
Adverse Effects of Lead

Neurologic Effects	Heme Synthesis Effects	Other Effects	Lowest Level Pb-B ($\mu g/dL$) Effect Seen
Deficits in neurobehavioral development (Bayley and McCarthy Scales); electrophysiological changes	ALA-D inhibition	Reduced gestational age and weight at birth; reduced size up to age 7–8 years	10–15 (prenatal & postnatal)
	EP elevation	Impaired vitamin D metabolism; Py-5-N inhibition	15–20
Lower IQ, slower reaction time (studied cross-sectionally)			<25
Slowed nerve conduction velocity			30
	Reduced haemoglobin; elevated CP and ALA-U		40
Peripheral neuropathies	Frank anemia		70
Encephalopathy		Colic, other GI and kidney effects	80–100

Source: MMWR 1988; 37 (32): 482.

The most common toxic effects of lead are summarized in Table 4.3.[63] In the peripheral nervous system, lead causes segmental demyelination. In severe cases, this can present as 'wrist drop' or 'ankle drop,' the visible evidence of extensor muscle palsies. At blood lead levels of 30–50 μg/dl, reduced nerve conduction velocities are often found. Lead penetrates neurons, altering ion-metabolism and inhabiting adenyl cyclase and other oxidative enzymes in the brain. Direct destruction of neurons and massive cerebral edema from increased vascular permeability in the brain are the basis for acute lead encephalopathy. The blood-brain barrier is more permeable to lead in the fetus and young infant.

Early damage to the kidneys is evidenced by aminoaciduria, decreased glomerular filtration rate and decreased tubular concentrating ability. Hyperuricemic gout and chronic renal failure can occur as late effects of lead exposure.

Lead affects the metabolism of the placenta and has been associated with prematurity, lower birthweights, and premature rupture of membranes. Lead can cross the placenta and accumulate in fetal tissues during gestation: Umbilical cord blood lead levels are nearly equal to those of maternal blood. Neuro-behavioural deficits attributed to lead have been documented in neonates born to mothers whose blood lead levels were within the normal range for women in industrialized countries.[64]

Screening tests to determine the extent of lead poisoning in a population must take into account physiologic principles. Because lead is not suspended in serum, but is transported by erythrocytes, lead levels must be measured in whole blood. This 'blood lead level' is the best measure of *recent* lead exposure. The blood lead level may not be elevated if lead exposure has occurred in the past because the lead will have been deposited in body tissues, primarily bone. In other words, the total 'lead burden' of the body may be high despite a low level of lead in the blood. Only sophisticated mobilization tests or direct measurement of lead in teeth or bone can indicate body burdens of lead.

Lead's inhibition of haemoglobin biosynthesis provides another opportunity for screening. The enzyme (ferrocholatase) required for insertion of iron into protoporphyrin is inhibited by lead. Protoporphyrin accumulates in red blood cells and can be measured by FEP (free erythrocyte protoporphyrin) or ZPP (zinc protoporphyrin) determinations. These tests can be performed on a drop of blood obtained from a finger prick. Measurements can be made with a portable fluorometer. However, distinguishing lead poisoning from other causes of anemia (iron deficiency, thalassemia) requires further tests.

Implications for prevention

- Because mental retardation, hyperactivity, and severe neurologic dysfunction can result from even a single episode of acute lead poisoning, prevention must be the highest priority in addressing the lead problem. Banning lead from gasoline, house paint, and cosmetics, avoiding lead-containing folk remedies, carefully removing lead paint from existing houses, substituting non-lead glazes for cookware, removing lead pipes from plumbing systems, and setting strict emission standards for industries using lead are important approaches.
- As new information has surfaced about the effects of low levels of lead exposure, criteria for diagnosing lead toxicity based on blood levels have been revised downward. For children, an elevated blood lead is currently defined by the US Centers for Disease Control as a whole blood lead concentration of 10 micrograms per deciliter (μg/dl) or greater. A WHO panel recommended a level of 20 μg/dl for the European Economic Community standard.[65]
- The groups at greatest risk for lead exposure include:

    a. pregnant women, because of transplacental transfer of lead to the foetus,
    b. industrial lead workers, because of the very high doses they can receive,
    c. infants and young children, because of their hand-to-mouth activity, increased GI absorption of lead, and vulnerability of their developing brain and nervous system to damage by lead.
    d. substance-abusing teenagers who inhale leaded gasoline.

- The best tests to screen for lead poisoning in a population—whole blood lead levels and erythrocyte protoporphyrin levels—reflect only recent exposures to lead. Other tests must be done to determine the total body burden of lead.

Ionizing Radiation

Nature of the problem

Since the discovery of both x-rays and radium in 1896, the sources of radiation exposure to human populations have multiplied. Increased mining, processing, transportation, storage, and disposal of radioactive materials has accompanied the growth of nuclear power plants, nuclear weapons production, industrial and medical uses of radiation.

Information on the adverse health effects of radiation has come from many different areas:[72-77]

- the nuclear explosions at Hiroshima and Nagasaki in 1945 produced an excess incidence of acute leukaemia for at least 20 years after exposure, atomic bomb survivors exposed before 20 years of age had higher relative risks of radiation-induced cancers (thyroid, breast, leukaemia) than victims who were older at the time of the bombings, infants born after in-utero exposures demonstrated microcephaly (small head size) and mental retardation;
- uranium miners suffered high rates of lung cancer from the inhalation of radon gas (a decay product of uranium), there is a synergistic effect between radon and cigarette smoking in promoting lung cancer;
- workers painting radium on self-luminous instrument dials developed oral cancers (osteogenic sarcomas of the jaw) and cancers of the mastoid sinus (from radon gas) after pointing their brushes repeatedly in their mouths;
- thyroid tumors have occurred among nearly all children from the Marshall Islands exposed to fallout from a nuclear weapons test in 1954, growth retardation has also been documented;
- medical misadventures with radiation produced unanticipated results: bone tumors developed in patients receiving radiation for ankylosing spondylitis, tuberculosis of the bone, and tinea capitis, thyroid cancers occurred in children who received radiation to their head and neck for 'treatment of a large thymus', liver and bone tumors occurred after thorium dioxide (Thorotrast) was used as a radiologic contrast medium.

The release of radioactive gases from the nuclear power plants at

Three Mile Island in Pennsylvania (1979) and Chernobyl, USSR (1986) created international awareness that radiation hazards are not limited to the threat of nuclear war. After Chernobyl, there were at least 26 deaths, 300 people hospitalized with radiation sickness, and nearly 100,000 people evacuated from their homes.[73]

Physiologic considerations

Ionizing radiation refers to gamma-rays, x-rays, alpha- and beta-particles, and high-energy neutrons. Gamma rays are high-energy electromagnetic waves similar to x-rays. Alpha particles contain two protons and two neutrons. Beta particles are high-speed electrons. What these particles/energy forms have in common is the ability to remove charges from, or add them to, electrically-neutral atoms and molecules. The altered electrical status (ionization) of biological molecules can change their function. For example, irradiation of DNA molecules can produce change or loss of a base, fracture of one or both chains of DNA, or cross-linking within the molecule. The altered genetic material can result in cancers or mutations, can remain latent, or can undergo enzymatic repair.

Radioactive chemicals follow the same biological pathways as their non-radioactive relatives. Iodine-131 is taken up by the thyroid like dietary iodine. Strontium-90 is incorporated into bone like calcium. Different organs and tissues have different sensitivities to radiation. Rapidly-dividing tissues are the most sensitive. This is why the earliest and most severe damage from acute, whole-body irradiation is seen in the gastrointestinal tract (esophagitis) and hematopoietic system (bone marrow suppression). It also explains the unique susceptibility of the foetus to radiation, since foetal tissues are rapidly proliferating.

The 'half-life' of a radioactive material is the time required for one-half of the radioactive element to decay into some other form. Strontium-90 has a half-life of 28 years; plutonium-239 of 28,000 years; iodine-129 of 16 million years. The half-life gives an idea of how long a radioactive material will represent a hazard in the environment.

Ionizing radiation can have adverse health effects through external or internal exposure. The impact of radiation on a person will depend on many factors:[78]

- total dose of radiation,

- rate at which the dose is delivered,
- type of radiation,
- physical characteristics (particulate or gas, particle size, lipid and water solubilities) and chemical composition of the radio-active materials,
- route of exposure (inhalation, ingestion, absorption through the skin),
- the nature and extent of tissue exposed (lung, skin, GI tract, thyroid, bone, testes, ovaries, brain),
- the age, sex, and immune status of the host.

Exposure to radon, for example, occurs through inhalation of the gas in uranium mines or in homes built over uranium-containing geologic deposits. Adverse health effects are caused by the 'progeny' of radon, two isotopes of polonium (214 and 218). They are in the form of minute, solid particles that can be retained in the lungs and tracheo-bronchial tree. They emit alpha-radiation, which penetrates a distance of no more than 70 micrometers into tissue. Therefore, radon exposure primarily produces cancers limited to the respiratory tract.[74]

Synergistic effects can occur when radiation is accompanied by exposure to other carcinogens. In patients treated for Hodgkins disease, for example, secondary cancers are far more likely to occur when patients receive a combination of chemotherapy and radiation than with either treatment alone. Uranium miners who smoked cigarettes (a well-demonstrated cause of lung cancer) had higher rates of lung cancer than their non-smoking co-workers.

Children have a greater risk of exposure to radioactive pollutants in soil because of their normal hand-to-mouth activity; in air, because their ventilatory rates are higher per kilogram of body mass; and in milk, because of their high dietary intake (the major route of radioactive iodine and strontium exposure from above-ground nuclear weapons tests was via cows' milk).

Children also are uniquely susceptible to health damage from radiation because their longer life expectancy than adults places them at increased risk of cumulative effects; their higher metabolic rates means thyroid uptake of I-131 is higher; open epiphytes and rapid bone growth make children vulnerable to bone-seeking isotopes like strontium and plutonium; cell proliferation within the brain, which continues for months after birth means radiation-induced CNS damage is possible.[72]

Implications for prevention

- There is no known 'threshold' or 'safe' level of radiation exposure. Therefore, exposures must be minimized, whether their source is medical diagnostic tests, radiation-related occupations, nuclear power plants, weapons tests, or environmental handling of radioactive wastes.
- The foetus and a young child are at most risk from radiation.
- Radiation limits (for population or occupational exposures), must take into account the types of radiation, chemical forms, routes of exposure, and host characteristics (age, sex, cigarette-smokers, pregnant women, etc.).

Pesticide Poisoning

Nature of the problem

Chemicals play a major role in a variety of pest control activities around the world, both in agriculture and in public health. More than

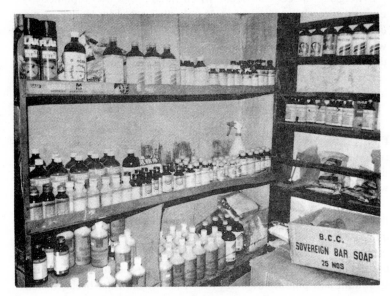

Photo 4.3: A wide variety of pesticides line the
shelves of this rural grocery store in Sri Lanka.

800 chemicals are currently used to control pests, weeds, plant diseases, and vector-borne illnesses.[80] The benefits of pesticides are seen in increased food production and reduced mortality and morbidity from such diseases as malaria, filariasis, and schistosomiasis. Yet, by definition, pesticides are poisons. Although pesticides must undergo toxicological evaluation before entering the market, pesticide misuse (both intentional and unintentional) is widespread over the globe. Between 400,000 and two million acute pesticide poisonings occur worldwide each year with an estimated 20,000 deaths.[80, 81] Most of the serious poisonings occur in LICs, where extremely toxic pesticides are sold in rural grocery stores along with other household goods (Photo 4.3). In some of these countries, pesticides are the leading causes of fatal poisoning (see Exercise 4).[82] The easy availability of aluminium phosphate in rural households has resulted in its among a large number of suicide cases. Several catastrophic events associated with pesticides have occurred since their introduction (Table 4.4).[83]

Table 4.4
A Brief History of Important Pesticide Events

1,000 BC	Sulfur used by the Greeks against household insects.
900 AD	Arsenicals are used by the Chinese.
1763	Nicotine, as crude tobacco, used as insecticide for plant lice.
1930's	10,000 people in the U.S. suffer paralysis from organophosphates used in making home-brewed liquor.
1939	Insecticide properties of DDT discovered by P. Muller.
1962	Rachel Carson's *Silent Spring* denounces DDT contamination of air and water.
1970	DDT banned first in Sweden because of ecologic effects.
1971–2	Organic mercury fungicide contaminates bread in Iran, poisoning over 5,000 people.
1976	Epidemic of malathion poisoning among 7,500 malaria workers in Pakistan.
1977	Dibromochloropropane (DBCP) restricted because of causing male sterility.
1984	Methyl isocyanate gas leak in Bhopal affects 150,000 people, killing 2,000.
1986	Over 1,000 tons of pesticides are spilled from a warehouse near Basel, Switzerland, into the Rhine River.

Adapted from Costa, L.G., reference 77.

Both the Food and Agricultural Organization (FAO) and the World Health Organization (WHO) evaluate pesticides for safety and efficacy.[84-86] A United Nations document, the International Code of Conduct on the Distribution and Use of Pesticides, provides guidelines on the availability, regulation, marketing, and safe use of pesticides.[87] However, promoting the safe use of pesticides through implementation of the International Code is difficult in LICs. Despite UN advice to the contrary,[88] warning labels usually do not mention the possible long-term adverse effects of the contents. Even when warnings and information about correct use appear on labels, such information is of no value to those rural people who are illiterate. Protective devices (masks, gloves, footwear, etc.) are frequently not designed for use in tropical climates. When protective devices of proven effectiveness exist, most farmers in LICs are too poor to buy them and wealthy landowners have little incentive to provide them to their employees. Agricultural workers are unorganized and usually politically powerless; they are usually desperate for work, and they are often migrants who lack the support of local communities.

Many governments in LICs have not been able to adequately control the manufacture or sale of highly toxic pesticides that are banned (or whose use is severely restricted) in HICs. For example, DDT and benzene hexachloride (BHC) account for three-quarters of the pesticides used in India; both are banned in the United States and most of Europe.[81] Factories for manufacturing banned pesticides are being transferred from HICs to LICs, or such pesticides are being manufactured in LICs under transfer-of-technology agreements. The leak of methyl isocyanate in Bhopal, India (where over 2,000 people died) was from a pesticide factory owned by a US corporation, Union Carbide Company. Lindane and gamma-BHC, which are banned in Japan and 19 other countries, are manufactured in Malaysia by a Japanese firm. Pesticide hazards are not restricted to LICs, however. In addition to agricultural workers, the general public in HICs are exposed to pesticides in the environment. Widespread contamination with the herbicide atrazine, for example, has been reported in surface water in the United Kingdom and in groundwater in the United States. Pesticide residues in foods, both domestic and imported, are a serious concern in many countries.[81]

PHYSIOLOGICAL CONSIDERATIONS

Many of the harmful effects of pesticides in man have been well documented, although the mechanism of action is known for only a minority of them.[89] They include enzyme inhibition (organophosphates and carbonates), pulmonary fibrosis and renal failure (paraquat, diquat), neurotoxicity (methylbromide and other halogenated hydrocarbons), male sterility (DBCP), impairment of coagulation (warfarin), and lung cancer (inorganic arsenic).[90]

The anticholinesterases are the best-studied pesticides in terms of toxic action. They include the organophosphorus compounds (e.g., bidrin, malathion, parathion) and carbamates (e.g., carbaryl or Sevin, propoxur or Baygon, Carbofuran or Lannate).[91, 92] They inhibit the enzyme acetylcholinesterase in both the peripheral and central nervous system. The result is accumulation of acetylcholine at receptor sites producing impairment of neurotransmission.[93, 94] Originally developed as chemical warfare agents, the anticholinesterases are now used in both agricultural and household pesticides. In acute poisonings, the severity of symptoms is directly related to the rate and degree of acetylcholinesterase inhibition. Some agricultural injuries may be the result of pesticide exposures that cause CNS effects such as dizziness, inattentiveness, muscular tremors, and disorientation. In severe poisonings, serum cholinesterase activity is often less than 10 per cent of normal and patients can exhibit hypotension, cyanosis, convulsions, and coma.

The chlorinated hydrocarbons, DDT, endrin, aldrin, dieldrin, hepatcholor, kepone, and others stimulate the central nervous system.[95–97] Acute toxic effects of endrin are tremors, delirium, seizures, coma and death. A dose of 0.25 mg/kg of endrin can produce convulsions. For months after an acute poisoning with dieldrin, patients can have hyperactivity, personality changes, and occasional seizures.[98] These compounds are stored in adipose tissue, metabolized slowly, and excreted in breast milk.[99] Samples of breast milk from Nicaraguan women have shown DDT levels 45 times greater than W.H.O. tolerance limits.[81] DDT metabolism and excretion is a very slow process, occurring over a period of years.

Long term effects that have been attributed to pesticides include cancers, stunted growth of children, congenital heart and limb deformities, blindness, deafness, and diseases of the liver and nervous system.[81, 100, 103] One study, for example, found a six-fold increased risk of non-Hodgkin's lymphoma among Kansas farmers who used certain herbicides (especially 2, 4-D).[81] Scientific studies of the chronic effects of pesticides are difficult to undertake. Even crude estimates of the types and amount of pesticides to which people are exposed are usually not available, serious outcomes, such as birth defects, are very uncommon, even when there is an increased relative risk, and associations between pesticides and ill-health are confounded by poverty, illness, and malnutrition.

Implications for prevention

- All nations should adhere to and enforce the international guidelines on pesticides and other hazardous chemicals, such as the International Code of Conduct on the Distribution and Use of Pesticides and the London Guidelines for the Exchange of Information on Chemicals in International Trade,

- Further research is needed on the long-term effects of pesticides. Results must be widely disseminated among agricultural communities and policy makers,

- Much more effort should be made to educate users in both HICs and LICS about pesticide hazards and application techniques,

- More comfortable masks and other safety devices suitable for tropical climates should be designed,

- Alternate technologies and methods—such as integrated pest management, multiple-crop farming, and biological methods of pest control—should be promoted to decrease reliance on toxic pesticides. Funding for research and demonstration farms needs to be greatly increased in both HICs and LICs,

- Stringent occupational and environmental laws are necessary in LICs to protect both workers and the community at large from catastrophes related to the manufacture of highly-toxic chemicals.[101] For example, chemical manufacturing plants should not be built in densely-populated areas.

- Each country should have a strict registration scheme which makes the more hazardous pesticides available only to highly-trained operators.[102]

SUBSTANCE USE AND MEDICAL CONDITIONS IN MOTOR VEHICLE CRASHES

Alcohol

The most widespread pharmacologic substance consumed by the public is alcohol. The world commercial production of alcoholic drinks grew from 824 million hl in 1965 to 1295 million hl in 1980. Beer was two-thirds of the total.[104] In the two decades prior to 1983, factory produced spirits increased almost 240 per cent in the LICs with the most rapid increase in Asia. In China, for example, beer production quadrupled between 1979 and 1983.[105] These figures are conservative estimates. They do not include spirits produced in the USSR; nor home-produced beverages, such as traditional fruit- and cereal-based alcoholic drinks in Africa, Asia, and Latin America, nor illegally produced alcohol.[106]

Driving skills deteriorate at blood alcohol concentrations over 50 mg/dl.[107] Between 30 and 55 per cent of fatal traffic crashes in countries as varied as Chile, Zambia, and the United States involve alcohol.[105] Each year in the US, about 40,000 people are seriously injured in traffic crashes involving alcohol.[108]

Alcohol is also a risk factor in suffocation deaths, especially those involving inhaled food particles, deaths in house fires (because of the strong association between alcohol and smoking), and deaths from hypothermia, recreational activities, adult drownings, air crashes, occupational injuries, and falls.[109] (During a nine-week strike in Norway that stopped delivery of wine and spirits to retail outlets, there was a marked decrease in injuries caused by falls).[110] Although the association is a complicated one, alcohol is a major risk factor for all forms of violence.[111]

Alcohol related morbidity and mortality is not limited to industrialized countries:

In Papua, New Guinea in 1979, there were 67 deaths per 10,000 registered vehicles, one of the world's highest death rates for motor vehicle accidents; a large proportion of these were attributed to drunk driving.[112]

In Swaziland, alcohol plays an important role in 60 per cent of homicide cases. Drunken driving cases are assuming alarming proportions.[110]

42 of the 46 countries in the world where beer consumption increased by more than 50 per cent between 1975 and 1980 are classified as developing countries. The production and distribution systems have now become so internationalized that any country that wishes to protect its population against unwanted inflows of alcoholic drinks needs some form of international collaboration.[113]

Alcohol's biological effects

At high doses, alcohol causes nonspecific depression of the central nervous system, orthostatic hypotension, and direct damage to gastric mucosa. Moderate doses cause depression of neuronal pathways that are usually inhibitory, resulting in nystagmus, reduced coordination, and behavioral stimulation. The effects of alcohol on higher brains functions are varied. Even at plasma concentrations well below the legal limit for driving in many countries,

> all psychometric measurements of co-ordination and reaction time are adversely affected by alcohol. As the plasma ethanol concentration rises, the first higher functions to be impaired are those most dependent on prior experience and learning, such as discretion and social modesty. At higher plasma concentrations, defects in memory, flights of ideas, and mood swings all appear.[114]

Many commonly used medications can adversely interact with alcohol. Acetaminophen and isoniazid, for example, increase the risk of liver damage. Barbiturates and benzodiazepines increase CNS depression. Contrary to popular belief, coffee is not a reliable antidote to the depressant effects of alcohol.[115]

Physiology of Alcohol

The time required for absorption of ethanol by the digestive system depends on the form in which the alcohol is consumed, and on the timing, nature, and quantity of food that is eaten. Alcoholic drinks that do not contain sugar (such as whisky and cognac) are absorbed more rapidly by the stomach and small intestine than drinks with added sugar (such as liquors). If food is eaten before or during alcohol consumption, alcohol's entry into the bloodstream can be delayed. Fatty foods in particular have this delaying effect. Alcohol consumed after fasting will diffuse throughout the body in about 30 minutes. If consumed while eating a large meal, diffusion may take several hours (Figure 4.8).[114]

After absorption in the upper part of the digestive tract, alcohol enters the bloodstream. Its diffusion area is virtually the same as that of water. Nerve cells equilibrate with the concentration of alcohol in the extracellular fluid. Their biologic function alters proportionately to the concentration of alcohol.

As long as the quantity being absorbed is greater than the amount metabolised, the blood-alcohol level rises. Alcohol's elimination from the body occurs mainly by the liver. The capacity of the body to break down alcohol is virtually linear: about 0.15 g/l per hour (the range is about 0.10–0.35 g/l per hour).

Many attempts have been made to predict blood-alcohol levels based solely on a person's body weight and anticipated beverage consumption. Several factors make precise predictions of peak blood levels difficult:

- The alcohol content of beverages such as beer can vary considerably, and this is not always indicated on the container,

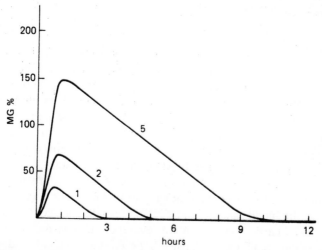

Figure 4.8: Typical curves for plasma ethanol concentration after ingestion of one, two, or five drinks. Both the peak levels and the duration in the body are increased with increasing alcohol intake. From Barnes, H.N. et al., *Alcoholism: A Guide for the Primary Care Physician,* p. 31. Copyright 1987 by Springer-Verlag, Inc., Heidelberg.

- Body weight is not a reliable indicator of the alcohol diffusion area. At the same weight, a more obese person will have a higher blood-alcohol level than a muscular person with little fat. This is because alcohol does not diffuse into fat. After consuming the same amount of alcohol, therefore, women have higher blood-alcohol levels than men of the same weight, since a higher proportion of female body weight is fat,
- The effect of food is difficult to assess. The sequence in which food and alcohol are consumed is very important in determining the peak alcohol level.

Problems also arise in trying to estimate blood alcohol levels in retrospect, such as after a motor vehicle crash. Given the almost linear kinetics of alcohol elimination, it would seem easy to calculate a person's alcohol level at the time of a crash based on knowing: 1) the blood-alcohol level after the crash, and 2) the time elapsing between the crash and collection of the blood specimen. However, such a calculation is not possible because of the variability in elimination rates among individuals and the uncertainty about when the peak alcohol level occurred.

Testing methods

The concentration of alcohol in a person's brain can be estimated by measuring alcohol levels elsewhere in the body, such as in blood or in expired air. A knowledge of the uses and limitations of alcohol measurements are important to the injury researcher studying risk factors, to the judge sentencing a convicted driver; and to legislators considering laws on drunk-driving. Two methods are now commonly used for legal purposes: blood testing and breath testing.

Blood testing for alcohol has greater precision than breath tests. It is performed by gas chromatography or enzymatic techniques. Because the blood sample can be retained, additional, confirmatory tests can be carried out. There are several disadvantages, however: considerable time often elapses between the incident and the sampling; venous blood is not as indicative of brain alcohol levels as arterial blood, haematocrit can influence the calculated concentration, the transport and storage of samples can alter the measured alcohol concentration. Breath tests, on the other hand, can be done with portable equipment (Photo 4.4), providing immediate

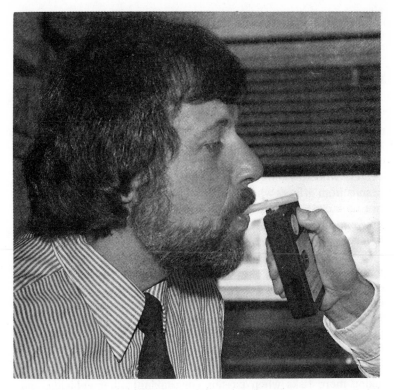

Photo 4.4: Accurate devices for measuring alcohol levels in the breath have become very lightweight and portable.

measurements. Breath alcohol levels closely approximate arterial blood levels. With frequent calibration, portable breath alcohol instruments are very accurate and reliable.[116] Not only have they become an essential component of drunk driving interventions, they are increasingly used in emergency departments to identify intoxicated injury victims.[117-119]

Epidemiological studies of alcohol and crashes

Many studies report the proportion of drivers involved in crashes who are 'under the influence of alcohol'. Because legal definitions and police procedures differ so widely, any study of the role of alcohol should specify the method used to detect alcohol; the alcohol level used to identify drivers as 'under the influence'; the total number of crash-involved drivers; and the number of cases in which a positive result was not obtained. It must be borne in mind that the driver of a vehicle may not have been the person responsible for the collision or injury.[120] For example, the intoxicated driver who causes a head-on collision may survive the crash, the non-intoxicated driver of the other car may be killed. The fatality would not be classified as alcohol-related if the only alcohol level measured is that of the deceased driver (as often occurs in data from medical examiners and coroners). Conversely, when alcohol levels are measured by breath tests, only drivers who can cooperate with the test will be included. Alcohol results from drivers who die, or who are rushed off to hospitals, will not be included in the reported cases. To analyze the association between alcohol and crashes, it is also critical to assess alcohol levels in a comparison group of drivers *not* involved in crashes.

Given these considerations, it is not surprising that statistics differ among epidemiologic studies. However, certain findings are very consistent: The risk of a driver becoming involved in a motor-vehicle crash increases as an exponential function of the blood-alcohol level. At blood alcohol levels above 1.5 g/l, the risk of crash involvement is tens of times greater than for a driver with no detectable alcohol. Some of the factors that may contribute to the increased risk of crashes among intoxicated drivers are: driving at higher speeds; taking more risks when passing (overtaking) other vehicles; and reacting more slowly and inappropriately to emergency situations. In test-track studies of drivers confronted by a police barrier located after a curve, braking and changing of course become progressively less efficient as the blood-alcohol level rises.

There is greater variability among individuals in their tolerance to alcohol. The driving performance of some people can be adversely affected by only one or two drinks. Legal limits for blood alcohol levels in drivers in different countries, therefore, range from zero to one g/l to no limits at all. The decision is based on political and socio-cultural factors, not scientific evidence.

Other Pharmacological Substances

Studies about pharmacological substances and crash risk are burdened by major practical constraints. There are often technical difficulties in detecting substances in blood, urine, breath, or saliva. Some tests are only qualitative and do not indicate the amount of drug consumed. Testing frequently requires complex devices which are expensive to purchase and difficult to maintain. For these reasons, studies are often limited to small population samples and therefore are of limited generalizeability.

Pharmacologic properties, such as a large volume of distribution and long elimination half-life, make positive blood or urine results difficult to interpret. Thus, merely demonstrating the presence of a substance in someone involved in a crash is not proof of its contribution to the event. Many teenagers smoke marijuana in the United States and many of them are involved in motor vehicle crashes. Is marijuana likely to increase the risk of a crash, perhaps by reducing driver attention? Or is an adolescent who smokes marijuana more likely to take all kinds of risks, including driving at recklessly and at high speeds?

Medications such as hypnotics, tranquilizers, and sedatives that interfere with mental alertness are likely to also interfere with driving performance. Here, again, there are enormous difficulties in studying the effects of these drugs on driving:

- because the drugs are prescribed within a fairly uniform dose range, it is not possible to establish a dose-effect relationship when studying crash risk,
- these drugs are used to treat morbid conditions (pain, anxiety, fatigue resulting from sleep disturbance, aggressivity, etc.) that may themselves be risk factors for impaired driving ability,
- behavioural effects of the drugs vary greatly between when the medications are first administered and later in the course of treatment,
- variations in individual response to a given preparation are common,
- there are a wide variety of preparations,
- it is difficult to assess the effect of combinations of preparations and the potentiating effect of alcohol.

To illustrate these points, consider the most commonly-used tranquilizers in industrialized countries, the benzodiazepines. Assume we conduct an epidemiologic study and find that a benzodiazepine is present in the urine of 10 per cent of persons involved in car crashes. Assume also that only 5 per cent of urines tests are positive among a comparison group of road users not involved in crashes. That crash-involved persons are twice as likely to have positive tranquilizer tests can be interpreted in several ways. The benzodia-zepines may cause drowsiness that leads to crashes. Alternatively, people who are prescribed a tranquilizer may be more irritable and high-strung, and therefore more likely to be involved in crashes. It is even possible that the type of people who use tranquilizers would be at greater risk of having a crash if they did *not* take the drug! In the absence of conclusive data, the best approach is to alert people taking these medications to the risk of drowsiness while driving or operating machinery.

Conducting studies of other psychoactive drugs—such as marijuana and the hallucinogens—is even more difficult. In addition to all the problems discussed previously, there is the added burden of il-legality; and the certainty that drug users differ in important be-havioral characteristics from non-users. Laboratory tests and driving simulation tests indicate that marijuana impairs attention and pro-longs the time required to make decisions, but does not increase risk-taking behavior. The effects vary considerably from person to person, and are related to previous experience with marijuana. Be-cause these tests are conducted with volunteers in artificial settings—not with actual substance users in actual driving situations—they must be interpreted with caution.

Medical Conditions

Rigid regulations that prohibit individuals from driving because of medical conditions are often arbitrary and discriminatory. A person with hypertension is at increased risk of a stroke. A recent heart-attack victim is at increased risk of a sudden life-threatening infarction. Yet, it would be wrong to prevent these individuals from driving a per-sonal automobile unless the increased risk was considerable, or at least greater than other risks tolerated by society. For example, many countries allow people to drive with a blood alcohol level up to one gram per litre, which makes them at least four times more likely to become involved in a crash than drivers with no alcohol in their blood. Research shows that accidents caused by the sudden physical or mental collapse of a driver are rare. Drivers with medical condi-tions, such as diabetes, epilepsy, hypertension, angina, that increase their risk of a catastrophic event almost always have time to stop without incident before losing consciousness. Scientific studies for estimating driving risks associated with medical conditions are rare; decisions must be made on an individual basis. In the case of a person with epilepsy, for example, the frequency of seizures and duration on medication have to be considered. An individualized approach is also important for persons with mental illnesses or physical disabilities (deafness, amputations, neurological disturbances affecting movement, etc.).

REFERENCES

1. DeHaven, H. 1942. Mechanical Analysis of Survival in Falls from Heights of 50 to 150 Feet. *War Medicine* **2**: 586–96.
2. Cairns, H. 1941. Head Injuries in Motorcyclists. *British Medical Journal* **4213**: 465–71.
3. Cairns, H. 1946. Crash Helmets. *British Medical Journal* **4470**: 322–3.
4. Planath, I., Nilsson, S. 1989. Testing and Evaluation of a Hybrid III Load Sensing Face. *Accident Analysis and Prevention* **21** (5): 483–92.
5. Foster, J. K., Kortge, J. O., Wolanin, J. F., Hybrid III. 1977. A Biomechanically Based Crash Test Dummy. In: *Proceedings 21st Stapp Car Crash Conference*, SAE 770938, pp. 957–1014.
6. Neathery, R. F., Kroell, C. K., Mertz, H. J. 1975. Prediction of Thoracic Injury from Dummy Responses. In: *Proceedings 19th Stapp Car Crash Conference*, SAE 751151, pp. 295–316.
7. Stapp, J. P. 1955. Effects of Mechanical Force on Living Tissues, I. Abrupt Deceleration and Wind Blast. *Journal of Aviation Medicine* **26** (4): 268–88.
8. Foust, D. R. et al. 1975. Cervical Range of Motion and Dynamic Response and Strength of Cervical Muscles. In: *Proceedings 17th Stapp Car Crash Conference*, SAE 730975.
9. Stalnaker, R. L., Mohan, D. 1977. Human Chest Impact Protection Criteria. *SAE Transactions*, SAE 740589, 2341–52.
10. Andersson, G. B., Ortengren, R., Herberts, P. 1977. Quantitative Electromyographic Studies of the Back Muscle Activity Related to Posture and Loading. *Orthop. Clin. North Am.* **8**: 85–96.
11. Cheetham, P. J., Sreden, H. I., Mizoguchi, H. 1987. The Gymnast on Rings—A Study of Forces. *Soma* **2** (1): 30–5.
12. Soutas-Little, R. W. et al. 1987. Biomechanical Analysis of the Athletic Shoe. *Soma* **2** (3): 18–22.
13. Paul, J. P. 1965. Bioengineering Studies of the Forces Transmitted by

Joints. In: R. M. Kenedi (ed.), *Biomechanics and Related Bioengineering Topics,* Pergamon Press, vol. II.

14. Lamoreux, L. W. 1971. Kinematic Measurements in the Study of Human Walking. *Bull. Prosth. Res.* 3: 10–15.

15. Mohan, D., Schneider, L. W. 1979. An Evaluation of Adult Clasping Strength for Restraining Lap-Held Infants. *Human Factors* 21: 635–45.

16. Kallieris, D., Schmidt, G., Mattern, R. 1989. Loading and Location of Rib Fractures in Simulated 90-Degree Car/Car Side Impacts with Post Mortem Human Subjects. 1989 International Conference on the Biomechanics of Impacts, 79–92. IRCOBI Secretariat, Bron, France.

17. Sacreste, J. et al. 1982. Proposal for a Thorax Tolerance Level in Side Impacts Based on 62 Tests Performed with Cadavers Having Known Bone Condition. In: *Proceedings 26th Stapp Car Crash Conference*, SAE 821157, pp. 113, 155–71.

18. Mathematical Simulation of Occupant and Vehicle Kinematics, SAE Publication, 1984, p. 146.

19. Ward, C. W. 1982. Finite Element Models of the Head and Their Use in Brain Injury Research. In: *Proceedings 26th Stapp Car Crash Conference*, SAE, pp. 71–86, 113.

20. Proceedings: Biodynamic Models and Their Applications. *Aviation, Space and Environmental Medicine* 49: 1, 1978.

21. MADYMO Applications, Version 5.0, TNO Road-Vehicles Research Institute, Delft, The Netherlands, 1992.

22. Bowman, B. M. et al. 1981. Simulation of Head/Neck Impact Responses for Helmeted and Unhelmeted Motorcyclists. *SAE Transactions*, 811029: 3318–44.

23. Fife, D., Ginsburg, M., Boynton, W. 1984. The role of motor vehicle crashes in causing certain injuries. *American Journal of Public Health* 74: 1263–4.

24. Eastman, J. W. 1984. Styling vs Safety: The American Automobile Industry and the Development of Automotive Safety, 1900–66, University Press of America, Lanham, MD.

25. Nahum, A. M., Melvin, J. 1984. Biomechanics of Trauma, Appleton and Lange, Norwalk, Connecticut.

26. Aldman, B., Chapon, A. 1985. Biomechanics of Impact Trauma. In: *Proceedings of the Symposium, Amalfi, 1983*, Elsevier.

27. King, W. F., Mertz, H. J. 1973. Human Impact Response: Measurement and Simulation, Plenum Press, New York.

28. An ounce of prevention: How Medical Professionals Can Work to Prevent Motor Vehicle Injuries. National Highway Traffic Safety Administration, 1981.

29. Holden, J. A., Christoffel, T. A Course on Motor Vehicle Trauma: Instructors Guide—Final Report/Users Manual. Report DOT/OST/P-34/86-050,

Office of University Research, US Department of Transportation, Washington, D.C., 20590.

30. 55 Speed Limit. IIHS Facts, Insurance Institute for Highway Safety, Washington, D.C., February, 1987.

31. Robertson, L. S. 1976. Estimates of motor vehicle seat belt effectiveness and use: Implications for occupant crash protection. *American Journal of Public Health* **66**: 850–64.

32. Nichols, J. L. 1982. Effectiveness and efficiency of safety belt and child restraint usage programmes: The safety potential of safety belts, child restraints, and programmes to promote their use. NHTSA, Washington, D.C.

33. Forster, J. H. 1984. When parents ask about car safety seats. *Contemporary Pediatrics*, November, pp. 59–72.

34. Bull, M. J., Bruner-Stroup, K. 1985. Premature infants in car seats. *Pediatrics* **75**: 336–9.

35. Air bags in perspective. 1993. Insurance Institute for Highway Safety Status Report **28** (11): 1–12.

36. Automatic passenger protection systems. 1984. *Pediatrics* **74**: 146–7.

37. Studies quantify effectiveness of air bags in cars. Insurance Institute for Highway Safety Status Report 1991; **26** (10): 1–2.

38. Mohan, D. et al. 1976. Air Bags and Lap/Shoulder Belts—A Comparison of Their Effectiveness in Real World Frontal Crashes. In: *Proceedings 20th Conference of the American Association for Automotive Medicine,* AAAM, Springfield, Illinois, pp. 315–35.

39. *Accident Facts: 1993 Edition.* National Safety Council, Itasca, IL, 1993, p. 68.

40. Mohan, D. 1986. Road Traffic Injuries in Delhi—Technology Assessment and Agenda for Control. *Proceedings of the International Seminar on Road Safety,* Indian Road Congress, Srinagar, pp. 93–125.

41. Hurt, H. H., Ouellet, J. V., Thom, D. R. 1981. Motorcycle Accident Cause Factors and Identification of Countermeasures, NHTSA, Washington, D.C.

42. Viano, D. C. Biomechanical interpretation of head injury mechanisms. In: Head Injury Mechanisms, Symposium Report, 30 September 1987, New Orleans, Louisiana, USA. Sponsored by AAAM and Volvo Car Corporation.

43. Gennarelli, T. A. Head injury biomechanics: A review. In: Head Injury Mechanisms, Symposium Report, 30 September 1987, New Orleans, Louisiana, USA. Sponsored by AAAM and Volvo Car Corporation.

44. Ommaya, A. K. 1988. Mechanisms and Preventive Management of Head Injuries: A Paradigm for Injury Control. In: 32nd Annual Proceedings Association for the Advancement of Automotive Medicine, AAAM, Arlington Heights, Illinois, pp. 360–91.

45. Motorcycle helmet issue. *Injury Prevention Network Newsletter,* Winter

1987–8; **4**: 1–15. Trauma Foundation, Building One, Room 400, San Francisco General Hospital, San Francisco, CA 94110.

46. Federal Motor Vehicle Safety Standards and Procedures for Customs Declaration and Certification of Imported Motor Vehicles. NHTSA, April 1985.
47. Robertson, L. S. 1981. Automobile safety regulations and death reductions in the United States. *American Journal of Public Health* **71**: 818–22.
48. Research Safety Vehicle. NHTSA, March, 1979. DOT HS 803 882.
49. Dole, C. E. 1988. Designing the cars of the future. *GEICO Direct Magazine*, Spring, pp. 19–23.

Scald Burns

50. Rogmans, W. H. J., Jackson, R. H. 1987. *Proceedings of the Conference on Prevention of Burns and Scalds*. Brussels, 27–8 November 1986, European Consumer Product Safety Association, Amsterdam.
51. Katcher, M. 1981. Scald-burns from hot tap water. *JAMA* **246**: 1219–22.
52. Feldman, K. W., Clarren, S. K., McLaughlin, J. F. 1981. Tap water burns in handicapped children. *Pediatrics* **67**: 560–2.
53. Feldman, K. W., Schaller, R. T., Feldman, J. A. et al. 1978. Tap water scald burns in children. *Pediatrics* **62**: 1–7.
54. Bergman, A.B. 1982. *Preventing Childhood Injuries*, Report of the Twelfth Ross Roundtable on Critical Approaches to Common Pediatric problems, Columbus, OH: Ross Laboratories.

Asphyxia

55. Choking and suffocation. 1991. In: Wilson, M. H., Baker, S. P., Teret, S. P., Shock, S., Garbarino, J. (eds), *Saving Children*, Oxford University Press, New York, Chapter 9.
56. Consumer Product Safety Commission Proposed Rules, Part 1501. *Federal Register* 1978; **43**: 47684–8.
57. Greensher, J., Mofenson, H. C. 1985. Injuries at play. *Pediatric Clinics of North America* **32**: 127–39.
58. European Consumer Product Safety Association (ECPSA). 1986. *Newsletter* **2** (4): 6.
59. Kravath, R. E. 1976. A lethal pacifier. *Pediatrics* **58**: 853–5.
60. Millunchick, E. W., McArtor, R. D. 1986. Fatal aspiration of a makeshift pacifier. *Pediatrics* **77**: 369–70.
61. Baker, S. P., Fisher, R. S. 1980. Childhood asphyxiation by choking or suffocation. *Journal of the American Medical Association* **244**: 1343–6.

Lead Poisoning

62. Needleman, H. L. 1980. *Low Level Lead Exposure: The Clinical Implications of Current Research.* Raven Press, New York.
63. Childhood lead poisoning—United States. 1988. *Morbidity and Mortality Weekly Report* **37**: 481–5.
64. Dietrich, K. N., Krafft, K. M., Bornschein, R. L. et al. 1987. Low-level fetal lead exposure effect on neurobehavioral development in early infancy. *Pediatrics* **80**: 721–30.
65. Landrigan, P. J., Graef, J. W. 1987. Pediatric lead poisoning in 1987: The silent epidemic continues. *Pediatrics* **79**: 582–3.
66. Dietrich, K. N., Berger, O. G., Succo, P. A. 1993. Lead exposure and the motor developmental status of urban six-year-old children in the Cincinnati prospective study. *Pediatrics* **91**: 301–7.
67. Sciarillo, W. G., Alexander, G., Farrell, K. P. 1992. Lead exposure and child behaviour. *American Journal of Public Health* **82**: 1356–60.
68. Landrigan, P. J. 1982. Occupational and community exposures to toxic metals: Lead, cadmium, mercury and arsenic. *Western Journal of Medicine* **137**: 531–9.
69. Coulehan, J. L., Hirsch, W., Brillman, J. et al. 1983. Gasoline sniffing and lead toxicity in Navajo adolescents. *Pediatrics* **71**: 113–17.
70. Guthrie, R. 1988. Prevention of lead poisoning in children—An issue for both developing and industrialized countries. *Pediatrics* **82**: 524–5.
71. Dolcourt, J. L., Finch, C., Coleman, G. D. et al. 1981. Hazard of lead exposure in the home form recycled automobile storage batteries. *Pediatrics* **68**: 225–30.

Ionizing Radiation

72. Berger, L. R. 1978. Child advocacy in the nuclear age. *Pediatrics* **61**: 802–3.
73. Balk, S. J., Neuspiel, D. R., Berger, D. K. 1986. Nuclear accident at Chernobyl: Implications for pediatricians. *Pediatrics* **78**: 1166–7.
74. Radon exposure: A hazard to children. *Pediatrics* 1989; **83**: 799–802.
75. Special susceptibility of children to radiation effects. *Pediatrics* 1983; **72**: 890.
76. Dreyer, N. A., Friedlander, E. 1982. Identifying the health risks from very low-dose sparsely ionizing radiation. *American Journal of Public Health* **72**: 585–8.
77. Miller, R. W. 1982. Radiation effects: Highlights of a meeting. *Journal of Pediatrics* **101**: 887–8.
78. Beebe, G. W. 1982. Ionizing radiation and health. *American Scientist* **70**: 35–44.

79. Effects of Nuclear War on Health and Health Services (Second Edition), WHO, Geneva, 1987.

Pesticides

80. Lotti, M. 1987. Production and use of pesticides. In: Costa, L. G. et al. (eds), *Toxicology of Pesticides: Experimental, Clinical and Regulatory Aspects.* NATO ASI Series, Volume H13: Springer-Verlag, Berlin.
81. Postel, S. 1988. Controlling Toxic Chemicals. In: Brown, L. R. et al. (eds), *State of the World 1988,* Worldwatch Institute, W.W. Norton & Company, New York, pp. 120–36.
82. Berger, L. R. 1988. Suicides and pesticides in Sri Lanka. *American Journal of Public Health* **78**: 826–8.
83. Costa, L. G. 1987. Toxicology of pesticides: A brief history. In: Costa, L. G. et al. (eds), *Toxicology of Pesticides: Experimental, Clinical and Regulatory Aspects.* NATO ASI Series, Volume H13: Springer-Verlag, Berlin.
84. Specifications for Pesticides Used in Public Health, Sixth Edition, World Health Organization, Geneva, 1985.
85. Joint FAO/WHO Food Standards Programme, Second Edition, 1986, Codex Alimentarius Commission, Codex Maximum Limits for Pesticide Residues, Codex Alimentarius, Volume XIII, CAC/VOL. XVIII-Ed. 2.
86. Environmental Health Criteria 104: Principles for the Toxological Assessment of Pesticide Residues in Food. World Health Organization, Geneva, 1990.
87. International Code of Conduct on the Distribution and Use of Pesticides. Rome, Food and Agriculture Organization of the United Nations, 1986.
88. Guidelines on Good Labelling Practice for Pesticides. Food and Agriculture Organization of the United Nations, 1985.
89. Hayes, W. J. 1982. *Pesticides Studied in Man,* Williams & Wilkins, Baltimore/London.
90. Davies, J. E., Enos, H. F. 1980. Pesticide monitoring and its implications. *Occupational Health and Safety,* March, pp. 68C–H.
91. Environmental Health Criteria 63: Organophosphorus Insecticides. World Health Organization, Geneva, 1986.
92. Environmental Health Criteria 64: Carbamate Pesticides. World Health Organization, Geneva, 1986.
93. Hayes, W. J. 1975. *Toxicology of Pesticides,* Williams & Wilkins, Baltimore/London.
94. Zwiener, R. J., Ginsburg, C. M. 1988. Organophosphate and carbomate poisoning in infants and children. *Pediatrics* **81**: 121–6.
95. Environmental Health Criteria 38: Heptachlor. World Health Organization, Geneva, 1984.

96. Environmental Health Criteria 83: DDT and its Derivatives. World Health Organization, Geneva, 1989.

97. Environmental Health Criteria 91: Aldrin and Dieldrin. World Health Organization, Geneva, 1989.

98. Rowley, L., Rab, M. A., Hardjotanojo, W. et al. 1987. Convulsions caused by endrin poisoning in Pakistan. *Pediatrics* **79**: 928–34.

99. D'Ercole, A. J., Arthur, R. D., Cain, J. D. et al. 1976. Insecticide exposure of mothers and newborns in a rural agricultural area. *Pediatrics* **57**: 869–74.

100. Schwartz, D. A., LoGerfo, J. P. 1988. Congenital limb reduction defects in the agricultural setting. *American Journal of Public Health* **78**: 654–9.

101. Baram, M. S. 1986. Chemical industry accidents, liability, and community right to know. *American Journal of Public Health* **76**: 568–72.

102. Plestina, R. 1989. Safe use of pesticides within the WHO programme. *Food Additives and Contaminants* 6 (Supplement No. 1): S15–20.

103. Mohan, D. 1987. Food vs Limbs—Pesticides and Physical Disability in India. *Economic and Political Weekly* XXII (13): A23–29.

Alcohol, Drugs, Medical Conditions

104. Walsh, B. M. 1985. Production of and international trade in alcoholic drinks: possible public health implications. In: Grant, M. (ed.), *Alcohol Policies*. WHO Regional Publications, European Series No. 18, pp. 23–44.

105. Heise, L. 1991. Trouble brewing: Alcohol in the Third World. *World Watch Magazine* 4: 11–18.

106. Smart, R. G. 1991. World trends in alcohol consumption. *World Health Forum* **12**: 99–103.

107. Simel, D. L., Feussner, J. R. 1988. Blood alcohol measurements in the emergency department. *American Journal of Public Health* **78**: 1478–9.

108. Drunk driving facts. National Center for Statistics and Analysis, National Highway Traffic Safety Administration, 1988.

109. Smith, G. S., Kraus, J. F. 1988. Alcohol and residential, recreational, and occupational injuries: A review of the epidemiologic evidence. *Annual Review of Public Health* **9**: 99–121.

110. Farrell, S. 1985. Review of National Policy Measures to Prevent Alcohol-Related Problems. Division of Mental Health, WHO, Geneva.

111. Fagan, J. 1993. Interactions among drugs, alcohol, and violence. *Health Affairs* **12** (4): 65–79.

112. Klaucke, D. N., The emerging problem of alcohol in developing countries. In: Risks Old and New: A Global Consultation on Health: Background Papers. Carter Center, Emory University, Atlanta, Georgia, April, 1986.

113. Sulkunen, P. 1985. International aspects of the prevention of alcohol problems: research experiences and perspectives. In: Grant, M. (ed.), Alcohol Policies. WHO Regional Publications, European Series No. 18, pp. 121–36.
114. Fox, A. W., Guzman, N. J., Friedman, P. A. 1987. The clinical pharmacology of alcohol. In: Barnes, H. N., Aronson, M. D., Delbanco, T. L. (eds), Alcoholism: A Guide for the Primary Care Physician, Springer-Verlag, New York, pp. 29–46.
115. Interactions of drugs with alcohol. 1981. *The Medical letter* 23: 33–4.
116. Giles, H. G., Kapur, B. M. 1991. Alcohol and the Identification of Alcoholics, Lexington Books, Lexington, Massachusetts.
117. Cherpitel, C. J. S. 1989. Breath analysis and self-reports as measures of alcohol-related emergency room admissions. *J. Slud Alcohol* 50: 155–61.
118. Gibb, K. A., Yee, A. S., Johnston, C. C. et al. 1984. Accuracy and usefulness of a breath alcohol analyzer. *Ann Emerg Med* 13: 516–20.
119. Gerberich, S. G., Gerberich, B. K., Fife, D. et al. 1989. Analyses of the relationship between blood alcohol and nasal breath alcohol concentrations. *Journal of Trauma* 29 (3): 338–43.
120. Zylman, R. 1971. Analysis of studies comparing collision-involved drivers and non-involved drivers. *Journal of Safety Research* 3: 116–28.

FURTHER READINGS

1. Nordin, M., Frankel, V. H. 1989. Basic Biomechanics of the Musculoskeletal System. Lea and Febiger, Philadelphia.
2. Injury biomechanics and the prevention of impact injury. In: Injury in America: A Continuing Public Health Problem. National Academy Press, Washington, D.C., 1985, chapter 4.
3. Wiktorin, C. H., Nordin, M. 1986. Introduction to Problem Solving in Biomechanics. Lea and Febiger, Philadelphia.
4. Organophosphorus insecticides: A general introduction. WHO, Geneva, 1986.
5. Mackay, G. M. 1981. Restraint systems, their use and effectiveness: A study. WHO, Geneva, ICP/ADR 035.
6. Sherman, J. 1988. Chemical Exposure and Disease: Diagnostic and investigative Techniques. Van Nostrand Reinhold, New York.
7. Needleman, H. L., Jackson, R. J. 1992. Lead toxicity in the 21st century: Will we still be treating it? *Pediatrics* 89: 678–80.
8. Prevention and care of motor vehicle injuries in the Caribbean. WHO, Geneva, 1984. IRP/ADR 216–25.
9. Benjamin, F. B. 1980. Alcohol, Drugs, and Traffic Safety. Charles C. Thomas, Springfield.

10. Ross, H. L. 1981. Deterring the Drinking Driver: Legal Policy and Social Control. Lexington Books, Lexington.
11. Alcohol, Drugs and Traffic Safety, Valverius, M. R. (eds), Box 5815, 102 48 Stockholm, Sweden. (A journal published four times a year.)
12. Problems related to alcohol consumption. Technical Report Series 650. World Health Organization, Geneva, 1980.
13. Jick, H., Hunter, J. R., Dinan, B. J. et al. 1981. Sedating drugs and automobile accidents leading to hospitalization. *American Journal of Public Health* **71**: 1399–1400.
14. Preventing lead poisoning in young children. Centers for Disease Control, Atlanta, October 1991.

5

Developmental, Behavioural and Socio-Economic Aspects

Age, gender, and the social environment influence the spectrum of injuries seen in a given community. The interaction between social and demographic factors is often complicated. The following sections hint at the complexity of behavioural and social factors contributing to the epidemiology of injuries.

FEMALE/MALE DIFFERENCES IN INJURY RATES

In most countries, males have higher rates of unintentional injuries than females at all ages (Table 5.1).[1, 2] Some, but not all, of these differences can be attributed to differences in *exposure*. For example, boys and girls have similar bicycle injury rates when adjustment is made for the amount of time the children spend riding their bicycles.[3] With playground slide injuries, adjustment for the amount of product use actually increases the relative risk of injury for boys compared to girls.[2] Studies of motor skills indicate that boys in later childhood and adolescence are at least as well coordinated as girls.[4] Therefore, the most likely explanation for higher injury rates among boys (when exposure is controlled for) is behavioural differences. In general, boys are more active, aggressive, and risk-taking than girls. Sex differences in injury rates among adults are greatly influenced by the gender-based division of labour. In rural areas of LICs, for example, hazardous activities such as chaff cutting and grain pounding are relegated to women, tractors are most often driven by men. In industrialized societies where both parents work outside the home, women continue to do most of the cooking, childcare, and housework with a predictable increase in the rate of certain domestic injuries, such as burns related to cooking.

Table 5.1
Male : Female Mortality Ratios for Accidents,
Poisonings, and Violence, Poland, 1978

Age Group	M:F Ratio
All Ages	3.4
Under 1 year	1.3
1–4	1.7
5–14	2.1
15–24	5.2
25–34	7.5
35–44	6.8
45–54	5.2
55–64	4.5
65–74	2.6
75+	1.3

Source: Adapted from Lopez and Ruzicka, reference 1.

Males are far more likely than females to be killed as a result of intentional violence, as illustrated by homicides in Thailand[5] and firearm deaths in the US (Table 5.2).[6, 7] Possible explanations are an increased use of alcohol, socialization of males to violence, and innate male aggressive tendencies.[8, 9] Yet women are frequently victims of non-fatal violence, such as sexual abuse, domestic assaults, and rape. In the United States each year, over 1.5 million women are treated for injuries related to abuse and over 1,800 women are forcibly raped

Table 5.2
Estimated Number of Firearm Deaths, United States, 1933–82

	Male	*Female*	*M:F Ratio*
All types	821,701	158,469	5.2
Suicide	408,769	69,112	5.9
Homicide	300,120	71,515	4.2
Unintentional	102,871	15,479	6.6

Source: Adapted from Wintemute, reference 7.

each day.[10, 11] Wife-beating is the most common form of family violence around the world and has been related to economic inequality,
male dominance in family decisionmaking, and restrictions on female
divorce freedom.[12]

CHILD DEVELOPMENT AND INJURIES

Physical, intellectual, emotional and social abilities change dramatically throughout the life cycle. Many of these changes have important
implications for both susceptibility to injury and the likelihood of
recovery from injury.[13] For example, many aspects of physical (and
physiological) development—such as motor skills, visual perception,
and tissue sensitivity determine a child's risk of injury:

- the ability to crawl, walk, and climb places different hazards
  in reach,
- improved fine motor skills allows toddlers to open bottles and
  medicine containers, contributing to poisonings,
- open epiphyses of bone subjects the child to growth plate
  fractures that can cause permanent disfigurement,
- growth and maturation of the nervous system increases susceptibility to neurotoxins,
- other immaturities of organ systems (GI, renal, pulmonary)
  may lead to increased absorption or impaired excretion of
  toxins,
- a thin epidermis and dermis increases the severity of burns
  and the absorption of chemicals,
- a large head-to-body ratio increases the risk of head injuries,
- decreased function of the apocrine sweat glands increases the
  susceptibility to heat stress,
- smaller airway size increases the danger of aspiration,
- smaller body proportions create a risk of head entrapment,
  diminished visibility to drivers in traffic, and reduced muscle
  mass to counteract dogs, refrigerator doors, and other hazards.

Lead poisoning illustrates the unique physiologic vulnerability of
children, where concern is warranted with blood levels greater than
10–15 micrograms.[14] Careful testing of children has demonstrated that
even children without symptoms of lead poisoning, but with elevated
body burdens of lead, may show deficits in intelligence, behaviour,

and school performance. (This topic is discussed in more depth in Chapter Four).

Limitations of intellectual development also place children at higher risk of injury through lack of knowledge and experience, lack of understanding of causality, undeveloped perceptual abilities to judge the speed of objects or to identify important risks amid competing stimuli, and poor judgement about risks and abilities. Equipment and machines, such as fodder cutters in India or grain transport wagons in the USA are not designed to protect children who are playing near them.[15–17] Modifications can be made to make equipment used around the home or on family farms safer, but only if the special needs of children are considered by the manufacturers.

Aspects of psychosocial development that impact on injury rates are the risk-taking behaviours of adolescents which contribute to alcohol and drug use, driving automobiles at high speeds, and engaging in dangerous recreational pursuits, and the normal exploratory behaviour of toddlers that attracts them to household chemicals, unattended medications, bodies of water, and lead paint.

Developmental considerations provide many explanatory insights into age-specific injury rates the prevalence of falls in toddlers whose ambulatory abilities are rudimentary, the high prevalence of pedestrian/motor vehicle injuries in children just starting school, the rise in motor vehicle injuries in children just starting school, the rise in motor vehicle occupant fatalities as teenagers enter driving age. Recognition of the developmental issues in injury causation also has implications for the reporting of injury data. Rather than providing injury rates grouped according to arbitrary age intervals (e.g., under 1 year, 1–4, 5–10, etc.), grouping data by developmental stages has much to speak for it. One such grouping, which incorporates aspects of physical, cognitive, and psychosocial development, would be:

- infants: under 1 year of age
- toddlers: 1–2 years
- preschoolers: 3–5 years
- early school age: 6–12 years
- teenagers: 13–18 years.

Age groupings are obviously culture-specific. They would be different in populations when there are important psychosocial differences, such as early age of marriage or employment. An example of guidelines for counselling families in HICs about injuries to children, based on developmental considerations, appears in Table 5.3.[18]

Table 5.3
Child Safety Counselling by Developmental Age

Age	Safety Topics
Prenatal and/or newborn	Infant car seats
	Crib environment
	Falls
	Faucet water temperature 120–130°F
	Bath: drowning, burns
2 months	Infant car seat
	Toys—avoid small, breakable, or cords
	Rolling and falls
4 months	Reaching and grasping objects, ingestions
	Infant furniture
6 months	Crawling and pulling up electric cords
	and sockets,
	Pots and coffee cups,
	Suitable texture foods
9 months	Give Ipecac, phone no. of Poison
	Control Unit
	Poison proofing
	Sharp objects
	Stairs
1 year	Child car seat
	Inquisitive walker and climber
Toddler to preschool	Yards and streets
	Tricycles
	Play equipment: set up and supervision
Early school age	Fire
	Bicycles, streets
	Car seat belt
	Swimming instruction
Preteen	Seat belt
	Traffic and bikes
	Swimming
	Educate in safety attitudes
Teens	Drivers education, seat belts
	First aid and CPR
	Sports
	Drug, alcohol, and smoking abuse

ACCIDENT PRONENESS, DISABILITIES
AND PSYCHO-SOCIAL STRESS

When otherwise healthy children seem to have more than their share of injuries, bruises, lacerations, burns, fractures, they are often said to be 'accident prone'. This implies that these children are predisposed to injury because of some identifiable trait, such as a gross lack of coordination or unusual impulsiveness. There is certainly no good data to suggest that individual children at high risk of injury because of specific behavioral characteristics can be identified prospectively. Most studies of psychosocial or behavioral factors and child injuries have been retrospective and/or poorly-controlled. A well-designed, prospective study which attempted to categorize children (150 seventh-graders) into high or low risk-taking groups failed to demonstrate an association between risk-taking and number of injuries over a 5-month period.[19]

There are reasons other than behavioral traits to explain why some children may suffer repeated injuries. 'Accident-prone' children may simply represent one end of a normally distributed curve, the upper five per cent of injury victims. Observed over a subsequent year, the number of injuries they suffer may be the same as an average group of children (in statistical parlance, regression to the mean would occur). Alternatively, there might be factors extrinsic to the child that are associated with repeated injuries. Several controlled studies have pointed to a relationship between childhood injuries and psychosocial stress, such as marital disharmony, financial problems, death or illness in close family members.[13, 21] A large scale study in Sweden found that children were much more likely to be accident repeaters, if their families were socially handicapped (receiving public assistance, known alcoholism, or were subject to the attention of the Child Welfare Board).[22]

Adverse family life events may increase the risk of child injuries because,

- parents may be preoccupied and therefore less likely to remove hazards from the environment and supervise children closely,
- children may become preoccupied and pay less attention to hazards,
- children may suffer guilt, loss of esteem, and helplessness.

They may then lose concern about their safety or act dangerously to distract their parent from arguments or sadness,
- psychoanalytic formulations may apply, such as counter-phobic antics of a child with haemophilia or fire-setting by a fatherless child.

Children with physical, developmental, or behavioural disabilities would be expected to be at higher risk for injuries. Mental retardation, neuromuscular disorders, sensory deficits (impaired hearing, vision, or tactile sensation), attentional deficit disorders (hyperactivity), autism, are all conditions likely to increase a child's exposure to hazards or decrease the child's capacity to cope with hazards.

HUMAN ERROR

Human beings are not perfect, it is impossible to be alert, aware, rested, attentive, responsive, and quick-acting at all times and under all circumstances. Injuries can therefore occur when there is a temporary imbalance between a person's performance level and the demands of the system in which the person is functioning. The demands can be reduced by design and environmental changes. For example, a sleepy automobile driver whose car swerves when he closes his eyes for a moment can escape harm if the highway has wide shoulders. If the shoulders are narrow or lined by ditches and trees (Photo 5.1) his car may crash. Similarly, a factory worker may be seriously injured if a co-worker forgets to turn off a machine. If the machine had an automatic shut-off device to immediately turn the power off when the machine was unattended, the injury could be prevented.

Behaviours called 'human error' are usually one of the following:

a) Aspects of normal behaviour: Being absent-minded at a factory after an argument at home; looking backward momentarily while driving when your child starts crying suddenly; stumbling over an unexpected toy on the floor and spilling a cup of hot tea on a child.

b) Unsafe behaviour as a result of faulty, uncomfortable, or unsafe designs or policies: Farmers in LICs will work at night with hazardous machines if electrical power is more expensive during the day; children will get their necks caught in slats on their

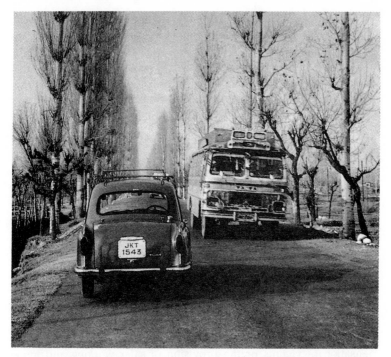

Photo 5.1: Narrow roads in many LICs are bordered by trees (for shade) and ditches (for drainage), allowing very little room for maneuvering. In HICs, roadside hazards include unforgiving concrete sign post and metal railings that can impale car occupants.

cribs if the distance between the slats is inadequate; a truck driver may run into a motorcyclist at night if the motorcycle's tail light is broken.

c) Unsafe behaviour and injuries resulting from lack of information: This is possible when a product is being used for the very first time and its special characteristics are not known. Product parts may have much sharper edges or points than expected, chemicals may be much more corrosive or reactive than expected, or a machine is much more powerful or moves much faster than expected.

d) 'Risk taking': Unsafe behaviour despite knowledge of the hazards involved: This is seen not only among teenagers, alcoholics, and psychologically-disturbed individuals, but also in perfectly normal adults who choose to engage in dangerous ativities like hang-gliding, mountain climbing, parachute jumping, etc.

The term 'human error' is often used by private businesses, government agencies, or other institutions to avoid responsibility for injuries or hazardous conditions. Consider the 'human errors' that might be involved when an elderly pedestrian is hit by a speeding truck:

- the pedestrian didn't judge the truck's speed accurately,
- the truck driver was going too fast,
- the police were not enforcing speed limits,
- the road designer failed to place speed control devices in the roadway,
- the traffic engineer didn't program the crossing lights with enough time for an old person to safely cross,
- the truck manufacturer didn't incorporate speed governors to limit maximum speeds,
- the government didn't provide adequate public transportation for elderly people.

By blaming the victims, larger social structures (such as municipal governments or employers of injured workers) can escape the compensation of victims or the provision of safer working and living environments. The insurance and legal systems are often engrossed in determinations of 'human error' in injury events. For purposes of injury prevention, however, the search for a single cause of an injury such as 'human error' is less useful than determining the constellation of factors that contributed to the injury.

INJURIES AMONG THE ELDERLY

As noted in Chapter One, older adults are becoming a larger proportion of the population of HICs each year. Elderly people have very high death rates due to injury (Figure 5.1).[23] Many of these deaths occur from home-related injuries such as falls, fires, and poisonings.[24] Pedestrian injuries are also an important cause of death approximately one-half of the pedestrian deaths in West Germany, for example, are persons over 65 years of age. Even a non-fatal but disabling injury can be catastrophic. The elderly victim may no longer be able to live alone, may become impoverished from medical and nursing care

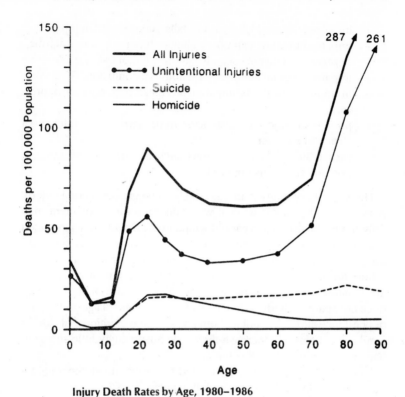

Injury Death Rates by Age, 1980–1986

Figure 5.1: Mortality data from the United States show three age peaks for unintentional injuries: Among infants, young adults, and the elderly. Injury death rates are highest for the oldest age group. From Baker, S.P., O'Neill, B., Ginsburg, M.J., Li, G., *The Injury Fact Book*, Second Edition Oxford University Press, New York, 1992, page 18. Copyright 1992 by Oxford University Press, Inc.

expenses, and may suffer steady declines in emotional and physical health.

Injury producing events are much more likely to occur among the elderly. Physical, sensory, social, and emotional impairments can reduce the capacity of the individual to cope with performance demands of the environment:[24-26]

- impaired mobility: difficulty crossing streets or controlling a fire,

- impaired vision: higher risk of falls and pedestrian injuries,
- impaired hearing: can't hear kitchen timers or house alarms,
- depression, fatigue, social isolation: alcohol use, suicide,
- impaired mental abilities: forgetfulness, confusion,
- multiple medications: impaired alertness, hypotension, depression,
- poor economic circumstances: hypothermia in winter, heat stroke in summer,
- associated medical conditions such as arrhythmias, strokes, postural hypotension, vertigo.

The severity of injuries are also likely to be greater among elderly persons. A 30 year-old woman who falls on an icy pavement may only have a bruise. A 90 year-old woman with osteoporosis, reduced muscle mass, and generally poor nutrition is likely to suffer a hip fracture that keeps her in the hospital for weeks or months.

Intentional injuries such as homicides, suicides, and physical abuse are a major problem for many elderly people. Intra-family violence does not spare individuals because of their advanced age. In fact, the dependence and vulnerability both physical and emotional of elderly family members may increase their risk. Surprisingly little research has been conducted on this topic.

Among the measures recommended to reduce non-intentional injuries among the elderly are the following:[26, 27]

- Falls: install nonslip strips in bathtubs and showers, handgrips next to the toilet and bath, rails on stairs, repair fall hazards, such as deteriorated stairways, loose carpets, and poorly-lit hallways, provide proper footwear;
- Burns: install smoke detectors in homes, reduce hot water heater temperatures to below 130 degrees to reduce scald burns, promote flame resistant clothing and sleepwear for older persons,
- Pedestrians injuries: improve traffic control and roadway design so that people with motor or sensory disabilities can cross streets easier (e.g., rest islands in middle of broad roads),
- All injuries: improve monitoring of medication use, especially of sedatives, promote physical fitness activities, provide low-cost, nutritious meals.

SOCIO-CULTURAL ASPECTS OF INJURY

Although little research has been done on the subject, socio-cultural factors play a major role in shaping the frequency and nature of injury events, and the intensity and success of efforts to prevent injuries. For example, the extent to which people make an effort to reduce injuries largely depends on their perceptions of how much control they have over their lives. In societies where individuals feel that they can influence decision making because organizations and governmental structures are viewed as responsive to citizens greater efforts are made to improve home, workplace and transportation safety. In most societies, the poor do not share these perceptions with the rich, therefore, they usually deal with most situations on an individual or family basis.

Secular, ethnic, and religious traditions also influence injury patterns. Allowing private citizens to own firearms with few restrictions is a tradition in the United States associated with an epidemic of violence.[6, 7] The homicide rate for young men in the United States is five to forty times greater than other industrialized nations.[28] Examples of injuries associated with religious traditions are burns from house fires caused by faulty wiring of Christmas tree lights, burns due to fireworks during India's 'Festival of Lights' (*Diwali*),[20] and head injuries of Sikhs who refuse to wear motorcycle helmets because their religious rules require them to wear turbans (they are exempt from helmet laws in India and the United Kingdom).

A well intentioned program in Nepal illustrates how socio-cultural influences can impact on prevention efforts:

> Most rural Nepali families cook over open fires. Not only does this use a great deal of increasingly valuable firewood, but children sometimes get burned playing near the flames. Also, the heavy smoke in the homes is thought to play a role in the high rate of acute respiratory illnesses. An inexpensive pottery stove (chulo) was devised that would reduce the amount of firewood needed for cooking, protect children from open flames, and vent the smoke outside the home (Photo 5.2).
>
> Introduction of the stove was not a resounding success, the chulos enclosed the fire, families could not longer heat more than one or two pots at the same time, requiring major changes in cooking patterns. Even the smoke was sorely missed, it had been vital for preserving foods and keeping the mosquitos away.

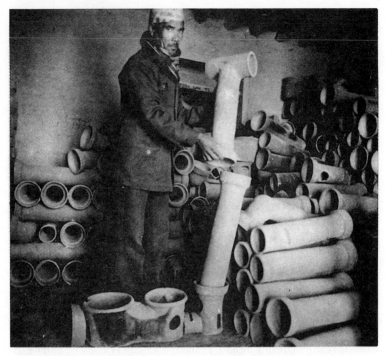

Photo 5.2: Clay stoves or '*chulos*' vent smoke from living quarters, decrease burns from open fires, and are more energy-efficient, reducing the amount of valuable firewood required for cooking and heating. Cultural practices and practical difficulties are barriers to their widespread acceptance in Nepal. (Photo courtesy of N. Thapa.)

Social and cultural factors also play a major role in defining and identifying injuries in specific populations. Shame, stigma, and legal consequences associated with intentional injuries such as 'dowry burnings' in India and suicides in most communities result in major under-reporting of these events. Even what constitutes an injury is subject to social and cultural interpretation. In the area of child abuse and neglect, for example, there is no universal standard for categorizing acts as 'abusive'. The definition depends on the age of the child, nature of the event, severity of the injury, relationship to the perpetrator, and other factors.[29] Social and cultural norms regarding abuse vary over time, among countries, and even within different communities.[30–32]

CHILD LABOUR AND INJURIES

In 1973, the International Labor Organization (ILO) adopted the Minimum Age Convention (Number 138) which established 15 years as the minimum age for employment. The 'minimum age' is actually a flexible one. For example, children 13 to 15 years of age can be employed in 'light work' (work which is not likely to compromise their health or school attendance). Also, workers must be at least 18 years old in particularly hazardous occupations.[33]

Estimates of the number of working children globally range from 50 to 300 million.[34] They include children working in carpet factories in Morocco, underground mines in Peru, match and fireworks plants in India, as domestic servants in Kenya, and shoe-shiners in Ecuador.[35] The majority of child workers, however, are in agricultural settings. Even in highly-industrialized countries, children on family farms or as migrant labourers are exposed to dangerous machinery and toxic chemicals. Each year in the United States, nearly 300 children die from injuries on farms and 23,500 suffer non-fatal trauma. While many of these deaths are not work-related, a large proportion of them are: the US Fair Labor Standards Act allows children of *any age* to be employed *in any occupation* on a farm owned or operated by their parent.[36, 37]

The conditions under which children work in the cities of many LICs are often highly dangerous to their health and safety.[38] Employers may be neglectful at best; physically, emotionally, and sexually abusive at worst. In small manufacturing plants, there is often inadequate ventilation, heating and lighting, long hours of work with inadequate rest periods and few days off each month, and monotonous tasks performed in one position. Crowded workplaces promote the spread of infectious diseases and lead to disasters when fires or other emergencies occur. Serious chemical exposures include lead from storage batteries, soldering, paint scraping and ceramics, cadmium from scrap metals and fertilizers, carbon monoxide from gas heaters and iron works, silica from quarries and glassworks, and asbestos from mines, construction work, and automobile brake linings. Physical hazards are numerous. Machines in LICs are often antiquated, with few built-in safeguards and irregular maintenance. There is usually a total absence of personal protective equipment (Photo 5.3). The work spaces themselves may be in danger of collapse or conflagration since few health, safety, fire or building regulations

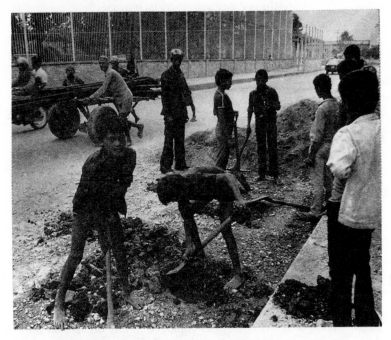

Photo 5.3: Children doing road work in Katmandu, Nepal wield picks and shovels without shoes or gloves for protection.

are enforced. For example, 85 per cent of child workers employed by manufacturing establishments in Bangkok worked more than eight hours a day.[39] Children who work as street hawkers or beggars wander for many hours amid busy road traffic.

There is scant epidemiologic data on injuries and other adverse health effects among child workers. Surveys underestimate both the number of child workers and the prevalence of injuries as child workers who have experienced severe injuries will not be present at the workplace, a phenomenon called the 'healthy worker effect;' employers are reluctant to allow researchers access to child workers, since child labour is illegal in most countries. The age of workers can be difficult to ascertain. Children may not know their birthdates or may lie about their age for fear of punishment by employers, parents or government officials.

The cultural, social, and economic determinants of child labour vary greatly among countries. Whereas a lack of educational facilities may be a very important factor in one country, social attitudes toward the role of women may be more important in another. In almost all countries, there are very different patterns of employment for boys and girls.

The medical sector can improve the lives of working children through both research and direct action. For each country, it is important to identify the nature and prevalence of hazards to working children. In what occupations or tasks are children engaged? What are the chemical, biologic, physical, and psychosocial hazards to which they are exposed? What are the demonstrable short- and long-term adverse effects of child labour in each country? By including questions about children's work activities as part of their medical history during both illness and well-child visits, physicians can provide valuable insights into child labour and its adverse health effects. By publicizing epidemiologic and clinical findings on the health dangers of child labour, the medical sector can raise national awareness and trigger community action. Governmental agencies, non-governmental organizations, and community support can be mobilized to enforce laws prohibiting child labour in especially hazardous occupations, and to improve living and working conditions for children in less dangerous occupations through medical, nutritional, educational, and social support programs.[40]

Labour for economic gain is not a developmental task of childhood. Ultimately, child labour must be totally abolished through direct social action, improved educational opportunities for children and adults, agrarian reforms, extension of family welfare measures, and sustained economic development leading to full adult employment.[41, 42]

REFERENCES

Child Development and Injuries

1. Lopez, A. D., Ruzicka, L. T. (eds). 1983. Sex differentials in mortality. Miscellaneous Series No. 4, Dept. of Demography, Australian National University, Canberra.
2. Rivara, F. P. et al. 1982. Epidemiology of childhood injuries. II. Sex differences in injury rates. *American Journal Diseases of Children* **136**: 502–6.

3. Waller, J. A. 1971. Bicycle ownership, use and injury patterns among elementary school children. *Pediatrics* **47**: 1042.

4. Angle, C. R. 1975. Locomotor skills and school accidents. *Pediatrics* **56**: 819–22.

5. Kanchanaraksa, S. (ed.). 1987. Review of the Health Situation in Thailand: Priority Ranking of Diseases. National Epidemiology Board of Thailand, Bangkok, April.

6. Rosenberg, M. L., Fenley, M. A. 1991. Violence in America. National Academy Press, Washington D.C.

7. Wintemute, G. J. 1987. Firearms as a cause of death in the United States, 1920–1982. *Journal of Trauma* **27**: 532–6.

8. Cherpitel, C. J. 1993. Alcohol and violence-related injuries. *Addiction* **88** (1): 79–88.

9. Choquet, M., Menke, H., Manfredi, R. 1991. Interpersonal aggressive behavior and alcohol consumption among urban adolescents in France. *Alcohol and Alcoholism* **24** (6): 381–90.

10. AMA Council on Scientific Affairs. 1992. Violence against women: relevance for medical practitioners. *Journal of the American Medical Association* **267**: 3184–9.

11. Mercy, J. A., Rosenberg, M. L., Powell, K. E., Broome, C. V., Roper, W. L. 1993. Public health policy for preventing violence. *Health Affairs* **12** (4): 7–29.

12. Levinson, D. 1989. Family Violence in Cross-Cultural Perspective. Sage Publications, Newbury Park.

13. Berger, L. R. 1981. Childhood injuries: Recognition and Prevention. *Current Problems in Pediatrics* **12**: 1–59.

14. Preventing lead poisoning in young children. Centers for Disease Control, Atlanta, October 1991.

15. Mohan, D. 1992. Design of safer agricultural equipment: Application of Ergonomics and epidemiology. *International Journal of Industrial Ergonomics* **10**: 301–9.

16. Field, B. 1980. Beware of flowing grain dangers. Pamphlet Number S-77, Purdue University Co-operative Extension Service, West Lafayette, Indiana 47907.

17. Swanson, J. A., Sachs, M. I., Dhalgren, K. A. et al. 1987. Accidental farm injuries in children. *American Journal Diseases of Children* **141**: 1276–9.

18. Feldman, K. W. 1980. Prevention of childhood accidents: Recent progress. *Pediatrics in Review* **2**: 75–82.

19. Padilla, E. R., Rohsenow, D. J., Bergman, A. et al. 1976. Predicting accident frequency in children. *Pediatrics* **58**: 223–6.

20. Mohan, D., Varghese, M. 1990. Fireworks cast a shadow on India's festival of lights. *World Health Forum* **11**: 323–6.

21. Husband, P., Hinton, P. 1972. Families of children with repeated accidents. *Arch Dis Child* **47**: 396–400.

22. Westfelt, J. N. 1982. Environmental factors in childhood accidents: A prospective study in Goteborg, Sweden. *Acta Paediatrica Scandinavica Supplement* **291**: 1–75.
23. Baker, S. P., O'Neill, B., Ginsburg, M. J., Li, G. 1992. The Injury Fact Book. Second Edition. Oxford University Press, New York, p. 18.
24. Hogue, C. C. 1982. Injury in late life: Part I: Epidemiology. *J Am Geriatrics Soc* **30**: 183–90.
25. Svensson, M. L., Rundgren, A., Larsson, M., Landahl, S. 1992. Accidents in the institutionalized elderly. *Aging* **4** (2): 125–33.
26. Rubenstein, L. Z., Robbins, A. S., Josephson, K. R. et al. 1990. The value of assessing falls in an elderly population. *Annals of Internal Medicine* **113** (4): 308–16.
27. Hogue, C. C. 1982. Injury in late life: Part II: Prevention. *J Am Geriatrics Soc* **30**: 276–80.
28. Fingerhut, L. A., Kleinman, J. C. 1990. International and interstate comparisons of homicide among young males. *Journal of the American Medical Association* **263**: 3292–5.
29. Berger, L. R. 1991. Protocol for the study of interpersonal physical abuse of children. *Maternal and Child Health*, WHO, Geneva.
30. Korbin, J. E. (ed.). 1981. Child Abuse and Neglect: Cross-Cultural Perspectives. University of California Press, Berkeley.
31. Giovannoni, J. M., Becerra, R. M. 1979. Defining Child Abuse. The Free Press, New York.
32. Gelles, R. J., Lancaster, J. B. (eds). 1987. Child Abuse and Neglect: Biosocial Dimensions. Aldine De Gruyter, New York.

Child Labour

33. Blanchard, F. 1983. Report of the Director-General. ILO, Geneva.
34. Child Labour: 1986. A Briefing Manual. International Labour Organization (ILO), Geneva.
35. Anti-Slavery Society Child Labour Series: Child Labour in Morocco's Carpet Industry (1978); Banerjee, S. Child Labour in India (1979); Searight, S. Child Labour in Spain (1980); Banerjee, S. Child Labour in Thailand (1980); Valcarenghi, M. Child Labour in Italy (1981); Ennew, J., Young, P. Child Labour in Jamaica (1981). Third World Publications, 151 Stratford Road, Birmingham B11 1RD England.
36. Cogbill, T. H., Busch, H. M., Stiers, G. R. 1985. Farm accidents in children. *Pediatrics* **76**: 562–6.
37. Rivara, F. P. 1985. Fatal and nonfatal farm injuries to children and adolescents in the United States. *Pediatrics* **76**: 567–73.
38. Shah, P. M., Cantwell, N. (eds). 1985. Child Labour: A Threat to Health and Development. Defence for Children International, Geneva.

39. Welfare and Development of Child Labour in the Manufacturing Industries. National Youth Bureau of Thailand, Office of the Prime Minister, Bangkok, 1987.
40. Research Methodologies and Techniques to Study the Health Problems of Working Children, 1988. *Maternal and Child Health*, WHO, Geneva.
41. Rodgers, G., Standing, G. (eds). 1981. Child Work, Poverty and Underdevelopment. ILO, Geneva.
42. Bouhdiba, A. 1981. Exploitation of Child Labour. U.N. Economic and Social Council, Commission on Human Rights, Document E/CN/4 Sub.2/479.

FURTHER READINGS

Child Development and Injuries

1. Langley, J., McGee, R., Silva, P. et al. 1983. Child behavior and accidents. *Journal of Pediatric Psychology* **8**: 181–9.
2. Bijur, P. E., Golding, J., Haslum, M. 1988. Persistence of occurrence of injury: Can injuries of preschool children predict injuries of school-aged children? *Pediatrics* **82**: 707–12.
3. Psycho-social factors related to accidents in childhood and adolescence. WHO EURO Reports and Studies, No. 46, Copenhagen, 1981.
4. Strategies de recherche action pour la prevention des accidents chez les enfants et adolescents. INSERM/WHO, Geneva, 1988. (English edition in preparation: Accidents in childhood and adolescence: the role of research).
5. Deschamps, J. P. 1981. Prevention of traffic accidents in childhood. EURO Reports and Studies 26. Regional Office for Europe, WHO, Copenhagen.

Elderly

6. Archea, J. C. 1985. Environmental factors associated with stair accidents by the elderly. *Clinics in Geriatric Medicine* **1**: 555–69.
7. WHO/ICSG Seminar on the Epidemiology of Falls in the Elderly: Summary Report. Injury Prevention Programme, WHO, Geneva, IRP/APR 216 m32 K, 9 April 1985.
8. Prevention of injuries to older adults: A selected bibliography. Centers for Disease Control, Atlanta, 1984.

9. Medical and social aspects of accidents among the elderly. WHO Injury Prevention Programme, Geneva, IRP/ADR 106–20(S), 1982.
10. The impact of demographic trends on health. *World Health Statistics Quarterly*, **40** (1). WHO, Geneva, 1987.

Child Labour

11. Annotated bibliography on child labour. ILO, Geneva, 1986.
12. All Work and No Play: Child Labour Today. Trades Union Congress, London, 1985.
13. Rodgers, G., Standing, G. 1981. Economic roles of children in low-income countries. ILO, Geneva.
14. Challis, J., Elliman, D. 1979. Child Workers Today. Anti-Slavery Society for the Protection of Human Rights. Quartermaine House Ltd., London.
15. Mendelievich, E. 1979. Children at Work. ILO, Geneva.
16. Taylor, R. B. 1973. Sweatshops in the Sun: Child labour on the Farm. Beacon Press, Boston.
17. Children at Work. 1987. Special health risks. Report of a WHO Study Group. Technical report series, No. 756, WHO, Geneva.
18. Workshop on research development in childhood accidents: Havana, 1984. WHO Injury Prevention Programme, Geneva, IRP/APR 216 m31K(S).

6

Translating Concern into Action

Data about injuries is useful only if it can be used to reduce suffering and deaths. This chapter reviews the conceptual framework for analyzing injury-producing events; the various approaches for reducing injuries; and the unique role of health personnel in injury control.

THREE FACTORS AND THREE PHASES OF INJURY

Consider the problem that many motorcycle riders suffer femoral fractures as a result of crashes. Describe the issue to the average person on the street, and the response is likely to be, we need to educate motorcyclists about how to drive more safely: whereas the surgeons response is 'Put more money into emergency medical services if you want to improve the outcome of highway injuries'.

Actually, the range of possible strategies for reducing motorcyclists femoral fractures is much greater than public education or emergency medical care. A valuable way to expand our thinking about options is through a model developed by Dr William Haddon. 'Haddon's Matrix' analyzes injuries according to three phases and three factors.[1] The phases of injury are chronologic; pre-event, event, and post-event. The three factors correspond to the host-agent model so well known to medicine and public health (Figure 6.1). The 'host' is the human factor the driver of a car, a pedestrian, or a child playing with fireworks. The 'agent' refers to the energy transmitting vehicle, motorcycle, pot of boiling water, threshing machine that can inflict an injury. The 'environment' includes both the physical environment (road, factory, residence) and the social environment (enforcement of speed limit laws, social acceptability of firearms).

Any type of injury can be analyzed by this model. Furthermore,

Factors

Phases	HUMAN	VEHICLE AND EQUIPMENT	ENVIRONMENT
PRECRASH			
CRASH			
POSTCRASH			

Figure 6.1: The 'Haddon Matrix'. From *To Prevent Harm*,
Insurance Institute for Highway Safety, Washington, D.C., 1978, p. 3.

the model can be used for analyzing both risk factors and possible interventions. Table 6.1 uses the model to categorize risk factors for burns among child workers in a textile factory. Table 6.2 illustrates strategies to reduce the burn injuries. For example, banning child labour is a strategy that is operative before any injury-producing event could arise (pre-event phase) and involves people (the human factor). Installing sprinkler systems in factories would reduce burn injuries if a fire broke out (event phase).

There is room for disagreement about where a particular risk factor or strategy fits in the matrix. For example, the sprinkler system can be considered an equipment factor or an environmental one. The purpose of the model is to stimulate a broad inquiry into risk factors and possible interventions, not to constrain ideas by decisions about where to place them in a matrix.

Table 6.1
Risk Factors: Haddon Model
Burns of Child Workers in a Textile Factory

	'Host' *Human*	*'Agent'* *Processes/* *Equipment*	*'Environment'*
Pre-event	Children easily fatigued, lack judgement about fire risks	Traditional dress (veils, saris) likely to go into flames	Factories poorly built and maintained
Event	Children panic when clothes ignite	No smoke alarms or sprinklers in factories	Crowded work spaces
Post-event	Adult supervisors put oils on burns	No sterile dressing available in factory	No running water inside factory

Table 6.2
Strategies for Injury Control: Haddon Model
Burns of Child Workers in a Textile Factory

	Human	*Processes/* *Equipment*	*Environment*
Pre-event	Prohibit child labour	Wear flame-resistant fabrics	Enforce electrical wiring codes
Event	Teach 'drop and roll' to child workers	Install sprinkler system in factory	Require at least 2 emergency exits from each room
Post-event	Teach first aid to supervisors	Provide first aid kits to each factory	Require water, bathroom facilities

Application of the model to the injury problem that began this section (femoral fractures among motorcyclists) is shown in Table 6.3.

Table 6.3
Reducing Serious Femoral Fractures in Motorcyclists

	Human	*Vehicle*	*Environment*
Pre-event	Educate motor-cyclists about safe driving	Install tires with excellent traction leather	Make roads less slippery and wet
Event	Wear pants made of heavy material	Provide leg guards on motorcycles	
Post-event	Teach the public how to splint fractures	Construct lighter-weight motorcycles	Improve ambulance services

CHAIN OF CAUSATION

In considering factors to include in the Haddon matrix, it is useful to think of a 'causal chain of events' leading to injuries. Each link in the chain is a potential point for injury prevention or control. This approach is contrasts with attempts to assign a single cause or prime determinant to injury events. For example, a motorcyclist dies from a head injury after being struck by a car at night. She had on a black leather jacket, made a left-hand turn when the traffic light was yellow, and was not wearing a protective helmet. The car that struck her was traveling at high speed. The official police report might have stated the cause of the collision as; driver of car did not see motorcyclist until too late to stop. Yet is there a single cause for this tragedy? The death might have been avoided if the motorcyclist had worn a bright-colored jacket, or used a safety helmet, or waited for a green light to make her turn, if the driver of the car had been traveling slower or had been more attentive, if the city highway department had installed brighter street lights at the intersection, if the police more vigorously enforced speed limits, or if excellent public transportation had obviated the demand for private vehicles.

A similar 'causal chain' can be constructed in the case of a young man who commits suicide while in jail (Figure 6.2). He began his day by going to a bar. He wanted to get drunk because he couldn't find a job and argued with his parents about money. Once drunk, he got

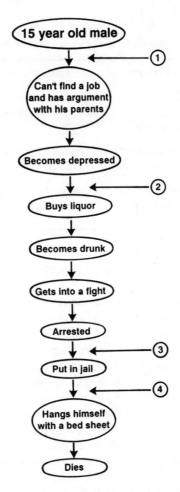

Figure 6.2: Chain of events leading to the suicidal death of an adolescent. Numbered arrows indicate several points for possible countermeasures (See text for explanation).

into a fight at the bar, the police were called, and he was arrested. Alone and depressed in a solitary jail cell, he used his bed-sheet to hang himself. Again, the many links in the causal chain in Figure 6.2 suggest opportunities for prevention: first create employment opportunities in the community for young people, second raise to 21 years the minimum age at which persons can buy liquor, third place intoxicated teenagers in the custody of their parents rather than in jail, and fourth if jailing an intoxicated or depressed adolescent becomes necessary, require suicide precautions such as close observation and removal of potentially lethal materials from the cell.

HADDON'S TEN STRATEGIES

Another major contribution of Dr Haddon to the field of injury control is his summary of ten *technologic strategies* for reducing the frequency and consequences of injury. These are:

1. Prevent the initial aggregation of the particular energy form.
2. Reduce the amount of energy aggregated.
3. Prevent the energy release.
4. Alter the rate or spatial distribution of release of the energy from its source.
5. Separate susceptible structures from the energy being released by means of space or time.
6. Interpose a material barrier to separate the released energy from susceptible structures.
7. Modify contact surfaces or basic structures that can be impacted.
8. Strengthen living or non-living structures susceptible to damage by the energy transfer.
9. Quickly detect and evaluate damage, and prevent its continuation or extension.
10. Carry out all necessary measures between the emergency period immediately following damage and ultimate stabilization of the process. Such measures include intermediate and long-term repair and rehabilitation.

How the ten strategies apply to different types of injury is outlined in Table 6.4.[2] Some of the examples are realistic to implement; others are more theoretical.

AUTOMATIC PROTECTION

The emphasis of Haddon's 'Ten Strategies' is on technologic modifications to reduce injuries. Trying to persuade people to act in self-

Table 6.4
Examples of 10 Basic Strategies for Reducing Injuries and Deaths

		Examples		
Strategy	Injury to motor vehicle occupants	Injury to football players	Injury by handguns
(1) Preventing the marshalling of potentially injurious agents or reducing their amounts.	Alternative travel modes; reduction in speed limits and speed capabilities of cars.	Fewer games; shorter quarters; speed restrictions in tackling drills.	Reduced production of handguns and bullets.
(2) Preventing inappropriate release of the agent.	Vehicle and road designs that simplify driver's task.	Playing surfaces that reduce likelihood of falls.	Locking up guns; eliminating motive for shooting (e.g., no cash)
(3) Modifying release of the agent.	Use of seatbelts, to decelerate occupant with vehicle.	Short cleats on shoes allowing foot to rotate, rather than transmit sudden force to knee.	Single-shot guns requiring reloading between firings.
(4) Separating in time or space or with physical barriers.	Restricting transport of hazardous materials to certain times and places; highway medians.	Limited contact practice drills; placing fixed structures further from field; face masks.	Bulletproof vests; bulletproof glass.

Strategy	Examples		
	Injury to motor vehicle occupants	Injury to football players	Injury by handguns
(5) Modifying surfaces and basic structures.	Airbags to spread forces over wide area of body; removing projections in car.	Padding outside of helmets.	Soft, doughnut-shaped bullets for target shooting (require less initial velocity and unlikely to penetrate humans).
(6) Increasing resistance to injury.	Therapy for osteoporosis.	Musculoskeletal conditioning.	
(7) Emergency response or medical care and rehabilitation.	Systems that route patients to appropriately trained physicians.	Personnel trained to recognize serious injuries, and physicians on call.	Occupational rehabilitation for paraplegics.

From: Baker, S.P., Dietz, P.E., Injury Prevention. In *Healthy People: The Surgeon General's Report on Health Promotion and Disease Prevention*, Background Papers, Washington, D.C., 1979.

protective ways is sometimes futile. Even when there are laws requiring individuals to wear seat belts or motorcycle helmets, the individuals most in need of protection (teenagers or people with alcohol problems, for example) are the ones least likely to comply. It is far more effective to provide automatic protection than to hope that people will behave in a safe way. Automatic approaches protect individuals without their having to perform some action or behave in a specific manner. For example, a person who chooses not to use her manual seat belt (or who forgets to buckle it) has no protection in the event of her car crashing. If there is an air bag in her car, however, it will inflate to protect her regardless of her state of mind, level of inebriation, or intelligence. Even staircases illustrate the principle of automatic protection. In walking down a flight of stairs, people usually pay attention to the first one or two steps to judge their configuration, then continue without watching their feet at every succeeding step. If stairs vary in length or height (Figure 6.3), falls are likely to occur, especially among the elderly and disabled. Uniformly-constructed stairs automatically protect everyone using them. Other examples of automatic protection are built-in sprinkler systems that are activated by smoke or heat, mechanical governors that limit the top speed of passenger trains, redundant cables in elevators, and

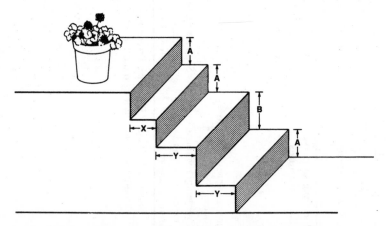

Figure 6.3: Variations in the length (X vs Y) or height (A vs B) of steps can lead to falls and subsequent injuries.

fences around swimming pools (so that parents do not have to supervise their children every minute to prevent them from drowning). Motor vehicle safety standards imposed by governments on automobile manufacturers are another example of automatic protection. Most of the standards are based on epidemiologic and biomechanical studies (see Chapter Four). Their effectiveness has been demonstrated in many countries over many years.

Injury countermeasures that offer automatic protection are the 'strategies of choice' for effective injury control. Automatic protection need not be prohibitively expensive, even in LICs. Examples of low-cost strategies are child-resistant containers for hazardous substances, children's chutes that are built into hillsides rather than above ground, and proposed designs for less damaging bus fronts (Figure 6.4)[3] and simple modification of farm devices (Photo 6.1 and Figure 6.5). Another example of an inexpensive approach, here involving traffic safety, arose during preparations for the 1985 Asian Games:

> When New Delhi was announced as the site for the games, a committee was formed to discuss traffic issues that might arise. Professor Dinesh Mohan, an injury prevention expert at the Centre for Biomedical Engineering, suggested that all three-wheeled, scooter taxis be painted yellow, rather than their traditional black. He said this would make the cabs more easily identifiable to tourists, but his primary goal was to reduce night-time collisions by making the taxis more conspicuous.

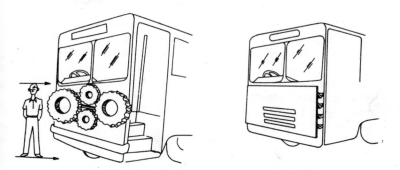

Figure 6.4: Two conceptual designs for reducing injuries when buses collide with pedestrians. On the left, discarded automobile tyres cushion the impact. On the right, a collapsible barrier serves the same purpose.

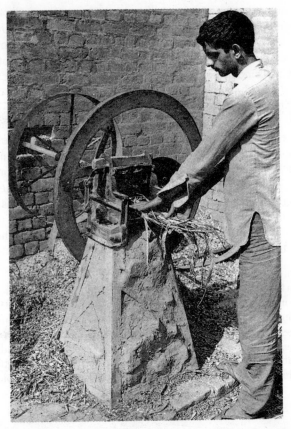

Photo 6.1: A chaff-cutter or fodder-cutter powered by an electric motor. Hands and fingers can be amputated if they become caught in the steel rollers that advance the fodder toward the rotating blades.

The taxi union objected to the expense. A compromise was reached—New Delhi three-wheeled taxis are now yellow on top, black on bottom! Regular four-wheeled car taxis are also yellow on top and black on the bottom half (Photo 6.2).

ARENAS FOR INJURY CONTROL: THE 4 E's

The ten technologic strategies involve *engineering*, i.e., changing the basic structure or function of injury-causing products to make them

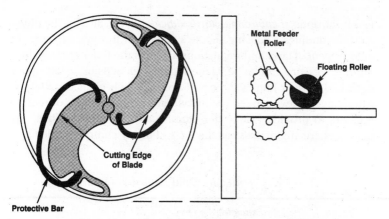

Figure 6.5: Simple modifications of chaff cutters could reduce amputations. *Left:* Protective bars ride in front of the cutting blades. *Right:* A smooth, floating roller serves as a warning that hands are approaching too close to the feeding rollers.

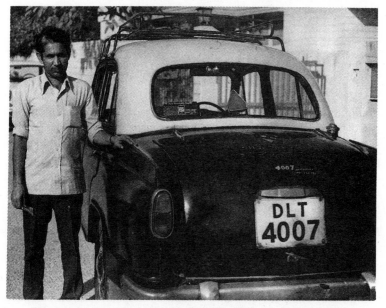

Photo 6.2: Only the top portion of New Delhi taxi-cabs are bright yellow; the rest of the car remains black. This cab also has an additional brake light mounted in the rear window, a device that dramatically reduces the likelihood of rear-end collisions.

less hazardous or *environmental modifications*, i.e., altering the physical surroundings. Changing people's behaviour through *education* or *enforcement* of laws and regulations also has the potential to reduce injuries. Persons can be persuaded to use seatbelts or install smoke detectors in their homes in order to reduce their chances of injury. Alternatively, laws can require individuals to use seatbelts or require builders to provide smoke detectors in all new homes. These approaches are summarized as the *4 E's* of injury control (Table 6.5).

Table 6.5
The 4 E's: Reducing Child Pedestrian Injuries

Approach	Examples
Engineering	Modify the front ends of vehicles so they will be less likely to hurt a pedestrian.
Environment	Improve night-time lighting of streets.
Education	Teach pedestrian safety to children in schools.
Enforcement	Increase arrests of drunk drivers.

Education

Community educational campaigns can inform people about unpublicized hazards and effective safety approaches, about the relative safety of similar products, such as automobiles[4] or household appliances,[5] and about laws and regulations that require public support and compliance. Although 'safety education' campaigns seem to make sense as a strategy, relying exclusively on education to reduce injuries is often ineffective.

Example 1: Household hazards

A paediatrician provided parents in his practice with detailed information about preventing household injuries such as burns and poisonings in children. The information was given verbally and in a booklet with daily safety advice. During a follow-up telephone call, the parents were asked if they had any difficulty child-proofing their home. When the homes were inspected during an unannounced visit, the number of hazards did not differ from homes where no safety information had been provided.[6]

Example 2: Television seat-belt messages

> Television advertisements were prepared by a panel of consumers and advertising experts to promote the use of seat belts. The ads were shown on a special cable network received by only certain families (intervention group). Comparison families did not see the special messages on their televisions. Observations of seat belt use were made at random locations in the community before and after the television campaign. The results: a slight decline in seat belt use by drivers from both intervention and comparison families![7]

Not only can educational efforts not be effective in reducing injuries, they may at times actually increase them:

Example 1: Drivers' education for teenagers

> Many secondary schools in the United States offer classes on driving motor vehicles. Students who pass these classes can obtain drivers licenses one to three years before teenagers who do not pass 'drivers education.' Financial cutbacks led to the cancellation of driving classes at several schools. The motor vehicle death rate for teenagers fell in those communities discontinuing the classes, compared with communities whose schools continued to offer them.[8]

Example 2: Fireworks safety pamphlet

> A ban on fireworks for personal use was proposed in one community. To prevent this from happening, the manufacturers of the fireworks suggested that their educational pamphlet would be adequate to prevent serious injuries. Included in the pamphlet was an illustration (Figure 6.6) showing a child making a bomb with gunpowder and a pipe![9]

Educational campaigns that target specific behaviors and whose messages are clear, culturally-appropriate, and widely disseminated can have an impact. Examples of specific messages are signs that tell construction workers to 'Wear Your Hard Hat' or billboards that warn car drivers to 'Wear Your Seat Belt.' Messages like 'Safety First!' or 'Drive Safely' are much too vague and consequently ineffective.

Even specific messages, however, do not guarantee a reduction in injuries, human behaviour is complex and often unpredictable:

> A media campaign in New Delhi had two goals: First, to discourage people from buying dangerous conical fountain fireworks during *Diwali*, a Hindu religious festival, and second, to get them to use cold water instead of traditional remedies if they were burned by fireworks.

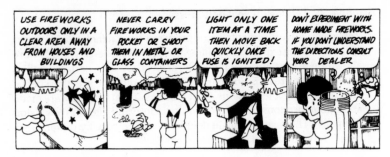

Figure 6.6: Panels from an 'educational' pamphlet distributed by fireworks companies. The last cartoon demonstrates how to build a pipe bomb!

A survey of emergency rooms found only a slight change in the choice of fireworks. The use of cold water, however, increased dramatically (Photo 6.3), from 5 per cent of burn victims in 1983 to 51 per cent in 1987.[10]

Enforcement/Regulation

Regulatory action can occur at a macro level (requiring car manufacturers to construct cars with safety specifications, building owners to have their elevators inspected by qualified engineers, employers to provide for the health and safety of their workers) or at an individual level (laws requiring car occupants to use seat belts or motorcyclists to wear helmets). The most effective regulations are those based on environmental and engineering approaches that have demonstrated value, but which might not be voluntarily implemented because of cost or inconvenience:

- Poison prevention packaging: Ten years after safety packaging of aspirin was required in the United States, deaths among young children from aspirin poisoning declined almost 90 per cent (Wilbur, C. J., unpublished).
- Inflammable fabrics standards: After sleepwear for children was required to be flame resistant, children with sleepwear-related burns declined from 17 admissions to one in five years at a burns unit in Boston.[11]

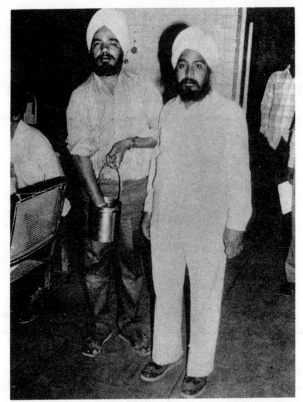

Photo 6.3: Burnt by fireworks, a man arrives with his friend
at a New Delhi emergency room, his hand still in cold water.
(Courtesy of D. Mohan, 1988).

- Motorcycle helmet laws: Over 90 per cent of motorcyclists
  wear helmets in the United States when they are required by
  law; less than 50 per cent do when laws are weakened or
  repealed. After repeal of the mandatory helmet law in Kansas,
  the incidence of head trauma to motorcyclists increased by 70
  per cent;[12] In New Delhi, it is mandatory for drivers of motorcycles to wear helmets but not for passengers. An observation-
  al study in that city[13] found over 90 per cent of drivers, but
  only 3 per cent of passengers, wearing helmets;
- Traffic speed limits: The association between crash fatalities

and the maximum speed limit was direct and consistent in Denmark (Figure 6.7);[14]

Motor Vehicle Crash Fatalities in Denmark Before and After Speed Limit Law Changes, 1970-82

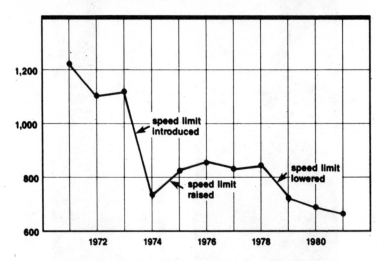

Figure 6.7: The number of people killed in motor vehicle crashes in Denmark varied with changes in the nation's speed limit. IIHS Facts, February 1987, p. 1. Reproduced with permission of the Insurance Institute for Highway Safety, Washington, D.C.

As potentially effective as a law may be, getting one passed is almost always a long and tedious process. Before undertaking the legislative route:

- Choose a problem that is important: consider the number and severity of injuries, the economic costs, and community concern about the issue,
- Have a goal that is well-defined and feasible,
- Gather the facts before recommending any action,
- Anticipate sources of opposition: Arguments that commonly arise in opposition to proposed laws are outlined in Table 6.6. There should be data, community surveys, government studies, published articles, to support your position,
- Build as broad a base of support for your position as possible.

Table 6.6
Common Arguments Against a Proposed Law or Regulation

- The problem is not that important.
- The proposed law won't work.
- It will cost too much.
- It is not legal (or constitutional).
- It is an undue burden on personal freedom.
- It is not feasible or enforceable.
- It is not popular with most citizens.
- If people would only take care of themselves and their families—by wearing seatbelts, supervising their children, etc., there would not be a problem.

Policy makers may not support laws or regulations to reduce injuries. The cost and inconvenience to industry of observing certain regulations may provoke opposition in a government that is trying hard to promote industrialization and employment. Other health and social issues compete for limited money and staff resources. Police may be more urgently required to supervise elections than to enforce traffic laws. Furthermore, passage of a law does not ensure its enforcement. The implementation of the law (or regulation) must be monitored and key decision-makers (police, legislators, judges, concerned citizens) must be informed of how the process is proceeding (or not) in the community.

A major barrier to effective regulatory action on an international level are the differences in regulations among countries. For example, the Organisation for Economic Co-operation and Development (OECD) is struggling with this issue in anticipation of a new European economic community in the 1990's. The Committee on Consumer Policy of OECD has undertaken a number of studies on product safety regulations among its member countries.[15] On a more global level, the United Nations expressed concern about the continued production and export of products that had been banned by one or more member governments because of their threat to human health or the environment. In 1982, the UN General Assembly requested the Secretary-General to prepare a list of products whose consumption and/or sale had been banned, withdrawn or severely restricted in their domestic markets. The resulting list covers pharmaceuticals, industrial and agricultural chemicals (including pesticides), and consumer products that are hazardous because of their chemical composition.[16] The World Health Organization and the UN Environment Programme have key roles in regularly updating the list. The second edition covers regulatory actions taken by a total of 77 governments on almost 600 products. Legal and bibliographic references, and brief explanatory comments, are included. A typical entry under 'Lead oxide and Lead salts' reads as given below.

Country: Denmark

Description of action taken/grounds for decision

> As a result of recorded cases of lead poisoning caused by excessive topical application, all pharmaceutical products containing lead compounds have been withdrawn.

A major incentive for the UN action was the recognition that many importing countries, especially LICs, did not have the information, expertise, and resources to keep up with developments in this field to protect themselves adequately.

Litigation is another aspect of enforcement. Manufacturers are less likely to sell defective products if there is a good possibility that they will be sued and suffer heavy financial losses. Toy makers, car manufacturers, and industrial corporations often have improved their operations after well-publicized lawsuits. In a landmark judgement, the Supreme Court of India has ruled that for industrial injuries, the amount of compensation and damages to be paid by the company will depend both on the actual damages and on the company's ability to pay. In LICs, where wages are extremely low, punitive damages are particularly important to encourage corporations to invest in worker and consumer safety.[17, 18]

COMPREHENSIVE PROGRAMMES

Proven and proposed countermeasures for reducing specific types of injuries in HICs and LICS are summarized in Table 6.7. Each of these measures is best implemented as part of a comprehensive approach. For example, a motorcycle helmet law seems like a 'pure' regulatory approach to an injury problem. An effective law, however, requires that dynamically-tested helmets are available, an engineering consideration. Also, extensive education is necessary: education of the police about the provisions of the law, of judges about the importance of enforcing helmet use, and of the public about the existence and desirability of the law. Arguing that regulations are 'better' than educational approaches misses the point that all the arenas—engineering, environmental modifications, enforcement, and education, are important in reducing injuries.

Table 6.7

Strategies for Injury Control in LICs and HICs

LICs	HICs
Motor Vehicles	
Mandatory motorcycle helmet laws for drivers and passengers.	Air cushions for both drivers for and passengers in all cars.
International safety standards for all motor vehicles.	Automatic shoulder/lap belts in all cars.
Speed bumps to reduce vehicle speed in populated areas.	Mandatory child safety seat laws.
Horsepower restrictions on motorcycle engines, imported and domestic.	Require helmets for bicyclists.
Reflectorized materials for clothing and for slow vehicles.	Lengthen stop-light signals to allow more time for pedestrians.
Widen road shoulders.	Strictly enforce speed and drunk-driving laws.
Support public transport over the import of private cars.	Extend public transport to reduce reliance on private cars.
Separate slow- from fast-moving traffic.	Lower speed limits.
Limit the sale of alcohol by taxes and other restrictions.	Limit the sale of alcohol by taxes and other restrictions.
Alter vehicle fronts to make them less damaging to pedestrians.	Mandate more strict car occupant crash-protection standards.
Fires and Burns	
Improve housing quality/safety for low-income people (e.g., provide low-cost, non-flammable materials).	Improve housing quality/safety for low-income people (e.g., enforce housing codes).
Replace high-pressure home cooking stoves with low-pressure, wick stoves.	Require smoke alarms in all homes.

LICs	HICs
Manufacture clothes with less flammable fabrics.	Manufacture clothes with less flammable fabrics.
Introduce inexpensive stands to stabilize bottle lamps.	Mandate self-extinguishing cigarettes; promote non-smoking.
Introduce chulos (enclosed ceramic stoves) to replace open fires.	Require hot water thermostats to be set no higher than 120° F.

Drownings

Provide covers for open wells.	Require fencing of swimming pools.
Increase inspection of ferries for safety.	Enforce 'no alcoholic beverages' regulations at public water recreation areas.
Improve local and regional flood control measures.	Enforce requirements for life vests on private boats.

Falls

Provide more stable climbing devices at construction sites (e.g., welded ladders).	Install window bars in apartments.
	Modify steps and stairs to reduce falls by the elderly and disabled.
Modify routines to reduce climbing of tall trees (see Exercise 5).	Install child barriers at stairs.
	Enforce safety standards for playground equipment and surfaces.

Poisonings

Design inexpensive, child-proof containers for kerosene, pesticides, etc.	Distribute Ipecac and poison information phone numbers to new parents.
Establish national and multi-national regulations for the manufacture and sale of pesticides.	Enforce regulations for lead content in paint, glazes, etc.
Establish national and multi-national regulations for the disposal of toxic wastes.	Reduce lead content of gasoline.

LICs	HICs
	Enforce regulations regarding disposal of industrial wastes.
Replace lead paint and glazes with non-leaded substitutes.	Increase inspection of car exhaust systems and home heating appliances to reduce CO exposures.

Intentional Injuries

Establish national and multi-national regulations for the manufacture, sale of pesticides.	Reduce the availability of firearms through restrictions on their import, manufacture and sale.

Agricultural Injuries

Install inexpensive safety features on fodder cutters and grain threshers.	Strictly enforce child labour laws.
Extend child labor protection to family farms.	
Provide increased educational opportunities for children.	Require roll-over protection for all farm tractors.

Non-Farm Occupational Injuries

Establish national and multinational safety standards for manufacturing machinery and industrial processes.	Increase the enforcement of in-dustrial safety standards through more frequent, unan-nounced inspections of mines and factories.
Eliminate child labour.	

Sweden's success in reducing childhood injuries, Thailand's National Safety Council, and the Consumer Safety Institute (CSI) of the Netherlands are examples of national programmes with a comprehensive approach to injury prevention.

Child Injuries in Sweden[19, 20]

Sweden has experienced a steady decline in injury death rates among children from birth to 14 years of age (Figure 6.8). The rates have fallen from 28 injury deaths per 100,000 children in 1953 to 12 in 1974

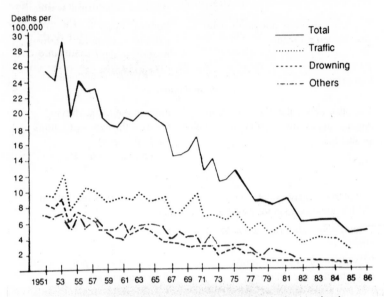

Figure 6.8: Sweden has experienced a steady decline in death rates among children from all types of injuries. From Berfenstam, R., Jackson, H., Eriksson, B. (eds), The Healthy Community: Child Safety as a part of Health Promotion Activities. Stockholm, 1987, p. 62. Folksam Insurance Group, WHO Regional Office for Europe, Child Accident Prevention Trust.

to 5 in 1985.[20] This dramatic decline has occurred despite the introduction of new technological hazards into the home, and reduction in adult supervision as more women work outside the home.

In 1953, pediatricians in the Swedish Society of Medical Sciences joined with the Red Cross and Save the Children Federation to form a Joint Committee for the Prevention of Childhood Accidents. Also represented on the committee now are government agencies (education, health and welfare, consumer policies, the Council for Children's Play), parents organizations, safety organizations (traffic, fire protection, lifesaving), and many professional bodies (such as physicians, nurses, and nursery school teachers). The aims of the Joint Committee are to encourage research about the patterns and causes of childhood injuries, to promote equipment and environments that will be safe for children, and to educate the public about child injuries and their prevention. An interim Working Group composed of two pediatricians and two pediatric surgeons, a representative each from the Red Cross, Save the Children Federation, the mass media, and insurance companies identify priorities and suggest activities to the member organizations.

Education of families about child safety is made possible by child-welfare nurses who make routine visits to the homes of babies and conduct group discussions with parents. Since 1938, Sweden has had a system of preventive child health centres. Over 95 per cent of young children are registered, providing extraordinary opportunities for both surveillance of health conditions and implementation of preventive programmes. Child-welfare nurses make routine visits to the homes of babies and conduct group discussions with parents.

The Joint Committee has promoted design changes and regulations through meetings with government agencies and manufacturers. As a result of these discussions, modifications have been made in home construction, interior design, household appliances, and leisure equipment. The National Board of Urban Planning issued child safety regulations for both homes and child centres. Windows accessible to children must be equipped with safety locks or barriers, glass in doors and windows must be strong enough to withstand children falling against them, doors to bathrooms must have securing devices that can be opened from the outside, storage places for chemical preparations and sharp household utensils must be equipped with child-proof locks, stoves must be constructed so that children are unlikely to come into contact with hot surfaces and cooking utensils.

The work of the Joint Committee is on-going, as new injury problems are identified and new approaches become available to address existing problems. The multi-disciplinary, community-based model for child injury prevention has been extended to all types of injuries.[21-23]

National Safety Council of Thailand

Since 1969, injuries have been the leading causes of death in Thailand, a nation with 50 million people. In 1983, there were over 33,000 deaths from injuries and nearly two million injury victims received medical treatment.[24] It is estimated that over half of the 700,000 disabled persons in Thailand became disabled because of traumatic injuries. The annual cost of motor vehicle crashes alone is between one and two per cent of Thailand's GNP.[25]

Unlike many LICs, Thailand had an over abundance of government agencies dealing with injury-related problems. At least 75 units under 12 ministries, including the Ministry of Public Health and the Departments of Highways, Land Transport, Police, Labour, and Industrial Works. The National Safety Council (NSC) was therefore established in 1983 as a central office to set priorities and co-ordinate government activities in the field injury. Sub-councils are devoted to traffic, occupational, agrochemical, public, and home safety. The work of the sub-councils is supported by committees for legislation and enforcement, education and training, public relations and public education, a National Safety Education Centre, and the National Accident Research Centre.

The NSC's President and Vice-President are Thailand's Prime Minister and Deputy Prime Minister, respectively. Council members include permanent secretaries of ministries and Directors-General of departments with direct authority for decision-making. The NSC offices are physically located on the grounds of the Prime Minister's office. Political support from Thailand's highest-ranking officials has lent enormous credibility and importance to the NSC's injury control activities.[25]

Consumer Safety Institute (CSI)[26]

The mission of CSI is to reduce home and leisure injuries. These are all defined as unintentional injuries other than traffic and occupational injuries. CSI operates PORS, the national surveillance system discussed in Chapter Two, conducts epidemiologic, biomechanical, and engineering studies, and serves as a consumer advocacy organization.

Research interests at CSI range from injuries among the elderly, children, and minorities, sports injuries, programme evaluation, including priority setting, cost benefit analysis, and outcome research. CSI also has developed testing methods and criteria for assessing the safety of electrical equipment, gas appliances, inflammable fabrics, children's articles, and architectural designs of both private and public buildings. Public awareness activities include a direct, toll-free consumer hotline and educational programmes on a national and regional level.

CSI has many co-operative relationships with national and regional agencies, universities, and non-governmental agencies. It works indirectly through the Ministry of Health of the Netherlands and directly with the Commission of the European Community, for whom it serves as the leading research institute in the field of home and leisure injury prevention. CSI is the responsible institute for the European Consumer Product Safety Association (ECPSA). CSI initiates most of ECPSA's international activities, such as its newsletter, conferences, and study reports.

THE ROLE OF MEDICAL PERSONNEL IN INJURY CONTROL

The importance of medical personnel providing direct curative services, including emergency care, to injury victims is obvious. There are, however, other roles for medical staff in the prevention and control of injuries: to identify injury hazards, record injury information, identify individuals at risk of injury, serve as community advocates, educate patients and families, and conduct injury research.[27]

Identify Injury Hazards

Medical personnel are in a unique position to identify important injury problems. Injuries that can be very damaging, but which occur infrequently, may be 'invisible' to most people in a community. Physicians, nurses, and other medical care providers see first-hand the entire spectrum of injuries in that community. They also have the opportunity to discover the details of how the injuries were inflicted.[28]

Example 1

Fireworks are sold and used in the United States almost exclusively during the July 4 celebration of independence. During one holiday, a pediatrician saw three children with injuries from fireworks: two children with burns to their hands and a third with an hyphema (bleeding in the eye). This led him to analyze the rate of injuries from fireworks in states which did and did not have strict laws regulating the types of fireworks that could be sold. The rate of injuries from fireworks was nearly 10 times less in states with strict laws.[29]

Example 2:

A 3-year old boy was brought to the emergency room in a coma. His parents found him on the floor of the bathroom next to an open bottle of mouthwash. The child recovered without complications after being treated for alcohol intoxication. A study of different brands of mouthwash found them to have higher concentrations of ethanol than many types of wine and beer.[30]

Example 3:

Dr Horace Campbell, a Denver physician, noticed in the 1960's that a number of people in car crashes suffered severe chest, head and neck injuries because the rigid steering shaft was pushed backwards and upwards into the driver. By bringing the issue to the attention of national safety organizations and the US Congress, he convinced automobile manufacturers to install collapsible steering columns in their cars. Similarly, Dr Paul Gikas (a professor of pathology) helped convince Congress to pass legislation mandating crash protection vehicle standards by showing slides of how sharp edges, pointed knobs, and other interior car design features caused serious, but preventable, injuries.[31]

Record Injury Information

As noted in Chapter Two, the most valuable information for designing preventive measures are details about the *circumstances of injury*. Yet medical records often contain only a minimal diagnosis ('fracture of forearm', '10 per cent burn to chest', head injury) and no details about how the injury occurred. Other data that is frequently missing, but which can also be of great value in studying injury problems in a community, are the *severity* of the injury and the *occupation* of the victim.

Identify Individuals at Risk of Injury

Because psycho-social factors (alcoholism, family stress, poverty) are associated with likelihood of injury, a social history should be part of every medical chart.[32] This means including such data as the persons with whom a child lives, any major social problems in the family (single parent, alcoholism), and any social service agencies already involved with the patient or family. Identifying patients at risk of injury also means considering possible intentional violence such as child abuse or self-inflicted injury so that help can be mobilized before more serious injury or death occurs. Another method for identifying patients who may deserve social support is to conduct regular chart reviews. A patient who frequently misses appointments, has multiple visits for injuries, runs away from home, or is absent a great deal from school raises concern about family stress. In such instances, the medical reviewer can notify an appropriate agency or person for follow-up. This may involve a children's protective team, an alcohol counselor, or a nurse or social worker to visit the patient's home.

Serve as Injury Control Advocates

Medical personnel usually have enormous respect in their communities. When they become involved in efforts to improve the public health, they have further credibility because there is no self-interest or hidden agenda to their activism. For example, automobile manufacturers may support mandatory seat-belt legislation in a country so that they will not be required to install automatic protection devices (which might lower their profit margins). When the medical society announces its support for laws requiring infants to be transported in car safety seats, there is no financial gain or obvious reward, other than the satisfaction of protecting children from harm.

The experiences of Dr Bent Sorenson, a surgeon working in a burn treatment unit in Copenhagen, are outstanding examples of how a physician can function as a community injury-prevention advocate:[33]

Each year in Copenhagen, between two and four children suffered severe scald burns at self-service laundries. The burns occurred when the children opened the doors of washing machines that were filling with hot water. They were splashed with water at a temperature of 80°C (176°F). To allow consecutive wash cycles to start with a minimum of delay between customers, the water temperature at the self-service laundries was much higher than in home washing machines.

Dr Sorenson contacted the government's Labour Inspection Service (LIS) about the problem. The LIS issued a regulation requiring that special safety locks be installed on the doors of front-loading washing machines 'if water of more than 65 °C can rise above the lower rim of the gate'. Since the regulation was issued, there has not been a single case of this type of scald injury.

Burn surgeons in Copenhagen began seeing many more children with mouth burns caused by electricity. They discovered that the circumstances of injury were almost always the same. Nearly all the victims were infants in the crawling stage. The children were playing on the floor while the mother was vacuum cleaning. The mother was interrupted in her work by something other than the baby, turned off the switch on the vacuum cleaner, but did not turn off the switch on the wall. In these injuries, the plug of the electric cord of the vacuum cleaner was broken and still live with current. A blue light sparked between the contacts on the plug, tempting children to examine it more closely by putting the plug in the mouth. Nearly all the broken plugs were manufactured by one firm. Convinced that only a few dangerous plugs were still in use, the firm offered to exchange them without charge for new, safe plugs. The media in Denmark advertised the exchange offer: the firm received 20,000 plugs. Twenty-three children were treated for electrical mouth burns in the five years prior to the campaign. In the five years after, only three children were treated with mouth burns, just one the result of a dangerous plug.

In 1971 in Denmark, some 3,000 people were treated for scalds due to coffee. Almost sixty per cent of them were burned when their coffee filters tipped over while they were brewing the coffee. The people of Denmark consumed nearly 50,000 tons of coffee—7 billion cups—that year. The most popular way of preparing coffee was to place the fresh grounds in a filter on top of an empty coffee pot. Then hot water was poured into the filter. The system was inherently unstable: the heavy filter and water-soaked coffee grounds sat above an empty container. Drs Asmussen and Sorensen published their findings and recommendations in a medical weekly. Their report was widely cited in newspapers, magazines, radio and television. They recommended that when brewing coffee, the pots should be placed in the kitchen sink and not on the kitchen table. They also urged people to discard their old filters and purchase a new, more stable type of filter (Figure 6.9). The physicians had previously approached the filter manufacturer. The company agreed to produce the new filter, but refused to withdraw the old filter from the market. Nevertheless, the number of coffee scalds in Denmark in the year after the campaign was reduced by two-thirds, from 3,000 victims to 1,000.

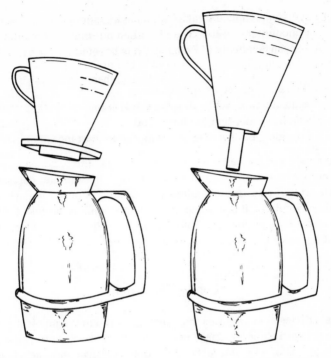

Figure 6.9: Scald injuries from coffee filters declined dramatically in Denmark when unstable filters (left) were replaced by more stable ones (right). Illustration based on a photograph in Sorenson, B., Prevention of burns and scalds in a developed country. *Journal of Trauma,* Volume 16, pp. 249–58, copyright by Williams and Wilkins, 1976.

Educate Patients and Families

The spectrum of health education delivered by medical personnel is very broad, from birth control information to nutrition advice to counseling about stress reduction. Because the amount of time that can be spent with individual patients is limited, and the tasks to be accomplished (history-taking, physical examination, charting, test ordering, supportive counseling, instruction about medications and follow-up) are numerous and important—the content of health education messages must be very selective. Only topics that are common and important causes of injury morbidity and mortality, and messages that have some chance of altering behavior, should be included in patient encounters. In the case of childhood injuries, for example, the American Academy of Pediatrics has targeted four areas of emphasis:

- the use of car seats and seat belts,
- installation of smoke detectors in homes,
- safe hot water temperatures, and
- providing bottles of syrup of ipecac to treat ingestions.

Obviously, the messages will vary according to the circumstances of difference communities and populations. For example, car safety seats are not relevant to families who are too poor to own an automobile. Similarly, it is a waste of everyone's time to discuss turning down the temperature of a hot water heater when the only means of heating water in a home is over an open fire.

Conduct Research

Most articles about injuries that have appeared in the medical literature concern clinical management rather than prevention. There are discussions of new diagnostic techniques, surgical approaches, and fluid therapies. The research questions most relevant to prevention, however, are epidemiologic, in that they involve groups of people rather than individual patients. Ready access to patient records allows physicians to analyze grouped data from their own patient populations. These local studies are important, because many injury issues are unique to certain communities. For example, injuries from falling out of the back of pickup trucks are common in Native American populations in the United States. Farm tractor injuries are frequent in agricultural areas. Childhood deaths involving firearms are concentrated in urban areas of the United States.

For readers interested in research, Exercise 7 outlines an approach to preparing a grant proposal. Assistance in writing proposals for injury control grants can be sought from individuals at local or national health departments or ministries, the WHO Global Programme in Injury Prevention, and schools of public health.

Even when medical staff are not directly involved in designing injury research activities, they can assist others carrying out such studies. They can advocate for the research with hospital committees and government agencies, facilitate access to medical records while insuring confidentiality, and participate in data-collection using specific forms and protocols.

BARRIERS TO MEDICAL STAFF INVOLVEMENT

The potential roles for medical personnel in the injury control field are clearly numerous and important. However, there are a number of reasons why physicians have not been more involved in injury control activities.

Injury/Disease Distinction

The disciplines of medicine and public health have never questioned that conditions as diverse as rabies, radiation sickness, and arthritis are within their realm of concern. Yet injuries have not been universally embraced by these disciplines, as if they are somehow very different. In fact, the distinction between 'injuries' and 'diseases' is a rather arbitrary one:

- A construction worker fractures his toe while using a jack hammer. Another worker is diagnosed as having tendinitis of the elbow from the chronic vibrations of the jack hammer.
- An operator at a nuclear power plant is burned severely when a fuel rod breaks open. A fisherman develops thyroid cancer 20 years after fallout from an above-ground nuclear test blanketed his boat.
- A child is bitten by a guard dog and requires 10 stitches to his leg. Another child dies of rabies after a bat bite.

In each of the above examples, the first victim we would say suffered from an 'injury', the second from a 'disease'. *Acuteness* is certainly a factor: the shorter the time from exposure to a hazard to physical effects, the more likely we are to call the resulting condition an 'injury' rather than a 'disease'. How arbitrary the distinction can be is illustrated by the following example:

In Iryan Jaya, Indonesia, several young children had been severely burned when they fell into open cooking fires. The children were tumbling into the fires because of sudden generalized seizures. A clinical and epidemiologic investigation revealed the cause of the seizures: cerebral cysticercosis, a parasitic disease caused by the larval form of the pork tapeworm, *Taenia solium.* Cysticercosis is endemic in many non-industrialized countries of the world. Treatment for cerebral cysticercosis has been largely limited to symptomatic control of seizures and increased intracerebral pressure, as well as surgery for ventricular shunting in hydrocephalus. In children, the disease commonly presents with single or multiple intracerebral cysts, often accompanies by diffuse or focal cerebral edema. Seizures and signs of increased ICP are the most common clinical manifestations in children.[34]

Burns, seizures, and a cerebral parasite, should the condition be described as an injury, neurologic condition, or disease? From a public health standpoint, the categorization makes little difference. Control of the disease still rests upon prevention by improvement in environmental and hygienic conditions.

Lack of Training

Medical persons are reluctant to promote approaches such as highway engineering or automotive designs in which they are not experts. In fact, injury research and prevention involves many disciplines other than medicine like sociology, psychology, statistics, public health, and engineering. Epidemiology, a discipline crucial to injury control, is still a very minor part of the medical school curriculum.

Many physicians also feel unequipped to approach problems on a community level. Actually, there are many analogies between the clinical approach to medical complaints and the community approach to injuries (Table 6.8). A person seeing a physician for abdominal pain, will undergo a history, physical examination, and perhaps special laboratory tests. A presumptive diagnosis will be reached, various interventions prescribed (e.g., medication, psychotherapy, and/or rehabilitative activities such as exercises), and a follow-up plan arranged. Similarly, when an injury problem like children falling from apartment windows is identified, available statistics and published articles on the problem can be reviewed (history), the apartments can be visited to observe the hazard directly (physical examination), the sequence of events leading to injury and available strategies reviewed, and interventions suggested (for example, using the '4 E's' described in Chapter Six). An evaluation of whether the intervention has been effective (follow-up) is an important component of any injury control activity.

Table 6.8
Analogy Between Clinical Approach and
Injury Control in the Community

Clinical	Injury Control
Chief complaint	Injury problem
History	Review of available statistics and relevant literature
Physical exam	Site visit
Special tests:	Targeted data-gathering/analysis:
Urine and blood	Medical record reviews
X-rays	Community surveys
Differential Diagnosis	Community Injury Analysis
Intervene:	Intervene:
Education (family, patient)	Education (community)
Medication	Regulation
Rehabilitation	Voluntary action
Counselling/Psychotherapy	Litigation
Follow-up	Follow-up

POISON INFORMATION CENTRES

The massive expansion in the use of chemicals, including pharmaceuticals, has created substantial risks from toxic exposures. Even in the low-income countries of the world, there is growing use of agrochemicals (pesticides and fertilizers), basic industrial chemicals, household products, and medications.[35, 36] Also, each country has a variety of natural toxins such as from snakes and other animals, plants, and fungi that could be hazardous to human health. The growing incidence of poisoning from chemical disasters, occupational exposures, unintentional ingestions, and suicide attempts have led to community-wide programmes for diagnosis, treatment and prevention.[37]

In addition to providing information and advice on poisonings to families and health professionals, a poison information centre (PIC) will often assist in implementing programmes to prevent poisonings; provide laboratory analytical services for poisonings, help manage poisoned patients, offer training in the field of poisoning prevention and control, develop plans for responding to major chemical disasters, and conduct research in poisoning prevention and toxicology. The medical disciplines supporting the creation of poison information centres include forensic medicine, pediatrics, pharmacology, emergency and intensive care. Many centres are connected both to a university hospital and to the public health service, and are supported at least partly by public funding.

Basic information on poisoning can be obtained from inquiries to the PIC, medical records from emergency rooms, forensic departments, hospitals, and occupational medicine clinics, medical and chemical publications, and literature from manufacturers and chemical importers. By routinely collecting this data for a community, the PIC can identify high-risk circumstances for poisoning, and mobilize community resources to address them. For example, a PIC can:

- alert responsible authorities to withdraw products from the market, or to require improved labelling or special packaging to reduce the risks of exposure to a toxic substance,
- contact manufacturers to encourage them to change product composition to a less toxic formulation or improve packaging and labelling on a voluntary basis,
- notify medical professionals of specific toxic risks, and
- inform the public about recognized community risks with respect to the use, transport, storage and disposal of specific toxins.

The methods employed for prevention of poisonings must be adapted to local situations and circumstances. Public education can occur through printed materials (brochures, leaflets, posters); mass media campaigns; and school-based educational programmes. (See the section on, Educational Approaches). Professional organizations, such as medical societies and pharmaceutical associations, often collaborate in poison prevention efforts.[38]

EMERGENCY MEDICAL CARE

The attention of the medical establishment in the area of injury control has focussed on the post-event phase: emergency transportation and medical care for injury victims.[39, 40]

Many of the approaches to civilian emergency care transport by helicopters and airplanes, training of skilled paramedics in the field, regionalization of trauma teams have come directly from military experiences. Since, at least, the reign of Napoleon, physicians have known that the mortality of trauma victims in wartime varies with the time to arrival at definitive care: the sooner a wounded soldier was treated, the better his chances of survival.[41] Of course, the urgency of needing medical attention depends on the primary problem. A person who suffers an out-of-hospital cardiac arrest must receive cardio-pulmonary resuscitation (CPR) in a matter of minutes to survive. An overdose of sleeping pills may not result in death for hours.[42]

In addition to rapid transportation, first aid has always been an important component of EMS. *First aid* may be defined as measures taken by lay people in cases of injury or sudden illness to prevent worsening and to maintain vital functions until qualified aid is available. Most first aid courses for the public include discussions of clearing the airway, the Heimlich maneuver, artificial respiration (mouth-to-mouth, mouth-to-nose, and manual compression), control of external bleeding, safe positions after injury (splinting fractures, neck stabilization), and prevention of shock. External cardiac resuscitation is often taught as well.

However, emergency medical services (EMS) consist of much more than first aid and rapid transport of victims to hospitals. EMS has been defined as:

> . . . a system which provides for the arrangement of personnel, facilities, and equipment for the effective and coordinated delivery in an appropriate geographical area of health care services under emergency conditions (occurring either as a result of the patient's condition or of natural disasters or similar situations). . . [43]

The components of EMS are numerous and complex (Table 6.9). Among the factors that need to be considered in designing an emergency medical system are:

Table 6.9
Elements of an EMS System

Public education
    recognizing emergencies
    first aid
    calling for qualified aid

Staffing and Training of emergency medical personnel
    firefighters, police, school personnel
    workers in hazardous occupations
    instructors in first aid practice
    communicators/dispatchers
    vehicle operators (drivers, pilots)
    hospital technicians (radiology, laboratory, blood bank, etc.)
    professional 'first responders' (paramedics, EMTs)
    nurses
    primary care physicians
    emergency medical specialist physicians
    medical administrators

Communication systems
    alarms
    telephone (toll-free, single number)
    medical consultation: computers, satellites

Emergency transport
    ambulances
    air transport
    radiotelephone

Administrative
    dispatching
    regionalization
    reimbursement
    setting standards
    planning and evaluation

Equipment, supplies, facilities
    stabilization
    transport
    hospital care

Data systems
    response time
    quality control
    financial
    improving care

Legal and political environment
   'Good Samaritan' laws
   medical care financing system

- type and frequency of injuries and acute illnesses,
- availability and distribution of health services,
- financial resources-population density,
- existing transportation facilities,
- geographic features,
- legal conditions.

Increasing attention is being paid to emergency management of large-scale disasters. Epidemiologic assessment and surveillance, effective use of personnel and supplies, co-ordination of international relief efforts, provision of adequate environmental health measures as well as the medical care for large numbers of casualties are major components of disaster planning.[44, 45]

In many countries, there is no legislation regarding emergency medical care. Where regulations exist, they often vary by local jurisdiction. Multiple government agencies and ministries are often involved at the national level and are not always co-ordinated. The mass media is infrequently used to promote awareness, except for disaster preparedness information in some countries. Emergency vehicles are more often available in cities than in rural areas, where even telephone communication may be limited or non-existent. When helicopter or fixed wing aircraft are used, they are usually police- or military-owned. Trauma data is usually collected by national health authorities rather than individual hospitals; there is little evidence that countries have attempted to use the data to modify or improve the emergency system or to conduct research.

An emergency medical system can be infinitely expanded. More money and resources can be invested in training, or communications, or equipment, or public education. Yet the cost of such services is enormous. The expense of maintaining a paramedic response team or a helicopter transport service for a region may be $1 million a year or more.[46] Also, even optimal emergency care cannot prevent many of the fatalities and permanent disabilities that result from trauma. One study in the northeast United States found that despite the availability of a sophisticated EMS system, 46 per cent of the people who died from motor vehicle trauma were dead at the scene and another 23 per cent died before reaching the hospital.[47] Recent studies also indicate that efficient emergency care can be provided without use of sophisticated technology. Use of medical anti-shock trousers, intravenous drips and portable ECG machines has not been found to make much difference in outcome. In some situations they can also be harmful.[48, 49] Obviously, emergency medical care is only one of many factors that are related to survival after an injury (Table 6.10).

Table 6.10
Factors Influencing Trauma Outcome

Age of patient

Sex of patient

Associated patient factors:

      medical conditions

      alcohol, drugs

Mechanism of injury

Body parts involved

Severity of injury

Pre-hospital care

Hospital care

Demonstrating which resources are the most cost-effective in terms of lives saved and morbidity prevented is an active area for EMS research. Other important issues deserving study are:

- What training should ambulance attendants be provided?
- What care should be delivered at the scene and what types of injury victims need to be transported immediately to a hospital?
- What kind of victims need to be treated at the nearest medical facility and who need to be taken to a centralized referral hospital?
- What is the eventual outcome—complete recovery, permanent disability, or death for victims who receive emergency care?

REFERENCES

1. Haddon, W., Baker, S. 1981. Injury Control. In: Clark, D., MacMahon, C. (eds), Preventive and Community Medicine. Little Brown and Co., 109–40.

2. Baker, S. P., Dietz, P. E. 1979. Injury prevention. In: Health People: The Surgeon General's Report on Health Promotion and Disease Prevention: Background Papers. Department of Health, Education, and Welfare, Washington, D.C., DHEW Publication No. 79-55071A.

3. Mohan, D. 1986. Road traffic injuries in Delhi: Technology assessment, agenda for control. Proceedings of the International Seminar on Road Safety, Sringara, Indian Roads Congress, New Delhi.

4. Injury and Collision Loss Experience: Cars by make and model. Highway Loss Data Institute. Annual publication.

5. Buying Guide Issue. Consumer Reports. Annual publication.

6. Dershewitz, R. A., Williamson, J. W. 1977. Prevention of childhood household injuries. *American Journal of Public Health* **67**: 1148–50.

7. Robertson, L. S. et al. 1974. A controlled study of the effect of television messages on safety belt use. *American Journal of Public Health* **64**: 1071–80.

8. Robertson, L. S. 1980. Crash involvement of teenaged drivers when driver education is eliminated from high school. *American Journal of Public Health* **70**: 599–603.

9. Berger, L. R. 1981. Childhood injuries: Recognition and prevention. *Current Problems in Pediatrics* **12**: 1–59.

10. Mohan, D., Varghese, M. 1989. Reducing burns from fireworks. *World Health Forum*.

11. McLoughlin, E., Clark, N., Stahl, K. et al. 1977. One pediatric burn unit's experience with sleepwear-related injuries. *Pediatrics* **60**: 405–9.

12. Russo, P. K. 1987. Easy rider—hard facts: Motorcycle helmet laws. *New England Journal of Medicine* **299**: 1074–6.

13. Mohan, D. 1983. A study of motorized two-wheeler use patterns in Delhi. *Indian Highways* **11**: 8–16.

14. 55 Speed Limit. IIHS Facts, Insurance Institute for Highway Safety, Washington, D.C., February 1987.

15. Product Safety: Measures to Protect Children. OECD, Paris, 1984.

16. Consolidated list of products whose consumption and/or sale have been banned, withdrawn, severely restricted or not approved by governments (second issue). United Nations, New York, 1987.

17. Teret, S. 1981. Injury control and product liability. *Journal of Public Health Policy* **2**: 49–57.

18. Swartz, E. M. 1971. Toys that Don't Care. Gambit, Incorporated, Boston.

19. Berfenstam, R. 1977. Learning from Sweden's experiences in preventing childhood accidents. *Pediatric Annals* **6**: 742–51.

20. Berfenstam, R. 1987. Some views on theory and practice in child accident prevention. In: Berfenstam, R., Jackson, H., Eriksson, B. (eds), The Healthy Community: Child Safety as a part of Health Promotion Activities. Folksam Insurance Group, Stockholm, pp. 61–5.
21. Bjaras, G. 1987. Experiences in local community activities in Sweden: The Sollentuna Project. In: Berfenstam, R., Jackson, H., Eriksson, B. (eds), The Healthy Community: Child Safety as a part of Health Promotion Activities. Folksam Insurance, Stockholm, pp. 167–73.
22. Schelp, L. 1984. Accident prevention within a primary health area. In: Berfenstam, R., Kohler, L., Methods and Experience in Planning for Accident Prevention. The Nordic School of Public Health, Stockholm, pp. 173–8.
23. Bergman, A. B., Rivara, F. P. 1991. Sweden's experience in reducing childhood injuries. *Pediatrics* **88**: 69–74.
24. Kanchanaraksa, S. (ed.). 1987. Review of the Health Situation in Thailand: Priority ranking of diseases. Bangkok, April.
25. Punyahotra, V. 1987. Accident control in Thailand. In: Proceedings of the Seminar on Accident and Injury Prevention Management at the Primary Health Care Level. Department of Medical Services, Ministry of Public Health, Bangkok.
26. Accident and injury prevention programme development. WHO, Geneva, 1988. IRP/APR 216 R 2667v, pp. 6–7.
27. Berger, L.R. 1982. The pediatrician's role in child advocacy. *Advances in Pediatrics* **29**: 273–91.
28. Berger, L. R. 1981. Childhood injuries: Recognition and prevention. *Current Problems in Pediatrics* **12**: 1–59.
29. Berger, L. R., Kalishman, S., Rivara, F. P. 1985. Injuries from fireworks. *Pediatrics* **75**: 877–82.
30. Weller-Fahy, T., Berger, L. R., Troutman, W. 1980. Mouthwash: A source of acute ethanol intoxication. *Pediatrics* **66**: 302–5.
31. An Ounce of Prevention: How medical professionals can work to prevent motor vehicle injuries. National Highway Traffic Safety Administration.
32. Berger, L. R., Kitzes, J. 1989. Injuries to children in a Native American community. *Pediatrics* **84**: 152–6.
33. Sorensen, B. 1976. Prevention of burns and scalds in a developed country. *Journal of Trauma* **16**: 249–58.
34. Gunawan, S., Subianto, D. B., Tumada, L. R. 1976. Taeniasis and cysticercosis in the Paniai Lakes Area of Irian Jaya. *Health Studies in Indonesia* **4**: 9–17.
35. Cardozo, L. J., Mugerwa, R. D. 1972. The pattern of acute poisoning in Uganda. *East African Medical Journal* **49**: 983–8.
36. St. John, M. A., Talma, T. E. 1982. A 5-year review of poisoning in children in Barbados. *West Indian Medical Journal* **31**: 121–5.

37. Guidelines for poison information centres: their role in prevention and response to poisonings. International Programme on Chemical Safety, September 1988.

38. Lovejoy, F. H., Caplan, D. L., Rowland, T., Fazen, L. 1979. A statewide plan for care of the poisoned patient. *N Engl J Med* **300**: 363-5.-

39. Schwartz, G. R., Cayten, C. G. 1992. Principles and Practice of Emergency Medicine, Third Edition. Lea and Febiger, Malvern.

40. Organization of emergency medical services. World Health Organization, Geneva, 1983 (IRP/ADR 218-24).

41. Cales, R. H., Trunkey, D. D. 1985. Preventable trauma deaths: A review of trauma care systems development. *JAMA* **254**: 1059-63.

42. Planning and organization of emergency medical services. EURO Reports and Studies Number 35, WHO, Copenhagen, 1981.

43. Praiss, I. L., Feller, I., James, M. H. 1980. The planning and organization of a regionalized burn care system. *Medical Care* **18**: 202-10.

44. Coping with natural disasters: the role of local health personnel and the community. WHO, Geneva, 1989 (ISBN 92-4-154238-1).

45. Nakajima, H., Should disaster strike—be prepared! World Health, January-February 1991; 2-3.

46. Urban, N., Bergner, L., Eisenberg, M. 1981. The costs of a suburban paramedic program in reducing deaths due to cardiac arrest. *Medical Care* **19**: 379-92.

47. Spain, D. M., Fox, R. I., Marcus, A. 1984. Evaluation of hospital care in one trauma care system. *American Journal of Public Health* **74**: 1122-5.

48. Wilson, A., Driscoll, P. 1990. ABC of major trauma, Transport of Injured patients. *British Medical Journal* **301**: 658-62.

49. Larsen, C. F. 1993. Prehospital Treatment of Injured and critically ill patients. Proceedings 12th World Congress of the International Association for Accident and Traffic Medicine, 1992. *Journal of Traffic Medicine Supplement* **21** (1): 192-202.

FURTHER READINGS

Translating Clinical Concern Into Action

1. Trinca, G. W., Johnston, I. R., Campbell, B. J. et al. 1988. Reducing Traffic Injury: A Global Challenge. Royal Australasian College of Surgeons, Melbourne.

2. First global WHO/NGO liaison meeting on accident and injury prevention. WHO Injury Prevention Programme, Geneva, 1985.

3. First interregional consultation on research development for injury prevention. New Delhi, 1985. IRP/APR 216m31R.

Role of the Medical Staff

4. Rivara, F. P. 1981. Injury prevention: The pediatrician as child advocate. *Developmental and Behavioral Pediatrics* 2: 160–2.
5. Claybrook, J. 1987. Stretching the physician's role: Giving priority to injury prevention. *Injury Prevention Network Newsletter* 5: 6–9.

Emergency Medical Services

6. Trunkey, D. D. 1993. Impact of violence on the nation's trauma care. *Health Affairs, Winter* 12 (4): 162–70.
7. Planning and organization of emergency medical services. WHO EURO Reports and Studies, No. 35, 1981.
8. West, J. G., Cales, R. H., Gazzaniga, A. B. 1983. Impact of regionalization: The Orange County experience. *Arch Surg* 118: 740–4.
9. Annotated bibliography of trauma care systems categorization and regionalization. *Ann Emerg Med* 1986. 15: 754–6.

7

Injury Control Interventions

MANIFESTO FOR SAFE COMMUNITIES

The First World Conference on Accident and Injury Prevention was held in Stockholm, Sweden, in 1989. More than 500 delegates from 50 countries participated. A fundamental premise of the meeting was that community-level programmes for injury prevention are the key to reducing injuries. At the conclusion of the conference, a 'Manifesto for Safe Communities' summarized important principles for injury control:[1]

local situations, unique resources, and the important cultural and socio-economic determinants of injuries must be recognized in order to develop safe communities,

- the public must be actively involved in planning and implementing community safety programmes,
- each government should formulate national policies and plans to create and sustain safe communities,
- priority should be given to injury prevention among vulnerable groups, such as children, the elderly, and the economically disadvantaged,
- a safe community involves not only the health and safety sectors, but also agriculture, industry, education, housing, sports and leisure, public works, and the media,
- national safety councils with multi-sectoral representation can support efforts at the community level,
- injury prevention programmes must incorporate existing community networks, such as mother and child clinics, school health education programs, and welfare services for the elderly.

This chapter explores important aspects of community based injury prevention—implementation, primary health care, community involvement, effective communication, funding—and concludes with examples of programmes in both HICs and LICs.

IMPLEMENTING A COMMUNITY INJURY PREVENTION PROGRAMME

A comprehensive, community-based approach to injury control links information and action in an on-going way. In practice, this involves the following steps:

1. Gather and analyze data on injuries in the community.
2. Select priorities for action: specific injuries and high-risk populations.
3. Formulate a community action plan: Choose intervention strategies that will work best in the target community given the available resources. Consider economic, social, cultural and political factors. Involve the community agencies and persons who will be most important in implementing the plan.
4. Train community members and support personnel, develop materials necessary for programme implementation.
5. Monitor and support the programme as it is implemented.
6. Assess the results and revise the action plan.

Community-based programmes in HICs are often established by public health agencies, or by non-governmental, non-profit groups specifically formed to address injury problems.[2, 3] In LICs, safety programmes in neighborhoods or villages are usually incorporated into existing primary health care activities.[4]

PRIMARY HEALTH CARE AND INJURY CONTROL

Primary health care (PHC) consists of promotive, preventive, and basic curative services usually provided outside of hospitals.[5] As described in the Declaration of Alma-Ata (produced at the 1978 International Conference on Primary Health Care):[6]

Primary health care is essential health care based on practical, scientifically sound and socially acceptable methods and technology made universally accessible to individuals and families in the community through their full participation and at a cost that the community and country can afford. It forms an integral part, both of the country's health system, of which it is the central function and main focus, and of the overall social and economic development of the community.

Primary health care has become a cornerstone of WHO's commitment to 'Health for All by the Year 2000,' a global strategy to achieve minimum standards of health throughout the world.[7, 8]

Several essential elements of PHC are relevant to injury control: education about prevailing health problems, maternal and child health care, prevention and control of locally endemic health problems, and treatment of common diseases and injuries. Efforts to incorporate injury control into PHC include the utilization of mother's groups and village craftsmen for primary health care efforts, coordination at the national level of a programme that includes injury surveillance, research, community and professional education, and development of appropriate technologies.

How readily injury prevention activities can be incorporated into the existing primary health care (PHC) system depends on a number of factors. Because village health workers have experience with medical subjects such as nutrition and family planning, principles of first aid can be learned and applied relatively easily. Acquiring skills in the mental health area (to reduce intentional injuries like homicide and suicide) and in non-medical injury subjects (such as road hazards and vehicle maintenance) may be more difficult. Similarly, because PHC workers spend much of their time with children and parents, targeting childhood and domestic injuries fits readily into ongoing activities. However, adolescents and young adult males, the groups most likely to suffer motor vehicle injuries, have not been included in many PHC programmes. Strategies to reduce injuries through technologic changes and regulations are not as familiar to the PHC system as health education approaches. Actions with a major economic impact such as requiring expensive repairs of motor vehicle defects are less likely to be implemented than low-cost approaches, such as teaching families how to treat minor burns with cold water. In summary, health education approaches that address domestic injuries, especially those involving children, will be the easiest to incorporate into existing PHC activities.[9]

TAILORING STRATEGIES TO LOCAL NEEDS

Strategies and technologies that are successful in HICs are sometimes unsuccessful or even counterproductive in LICs. Approaches must be tailored to the economic, social, cultural, political, geographic, and climatic conditions of the communities in which they will be implemented. Examples are:

- using local materials for basic prevention and first aid, bamboo for building stretchers and splinting fractures, textiles for head protection, neck collars, arm slings, and sunburn protection,
- substituting wick stoves (Photo 7.1) for pressurized stoves (Photo 7.2) that can explode,

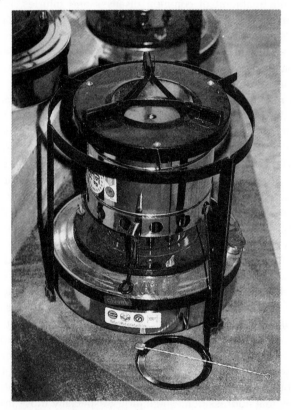

Photo 7.1: A low-pressure, multiple-wick, kerosene stove
Pressurized stoves—shown in Photo 7.2—frequently explode.

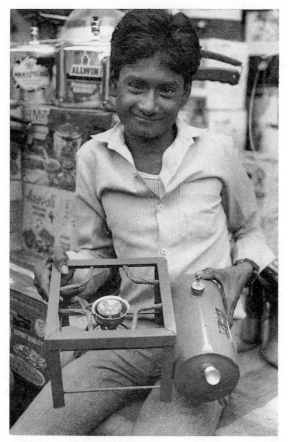

Photo 7.2: Pressurized kerosene stoves are widespread in LICs.

- supporting kerosene lamps on a stable base (Figure 7.1) to reduce fires and burns from spilled kerosene,
- installing 'speed breakers' to reduce motor vehicle speed in populated areas (Photo 7.3),
- tying loose clothing closer to the body when working near machinery (Photo 7.4),
- placing grass or sand beneath children's play equipment (Photo 7.5),
- working in teams rather than as individuals (Photo 7.6),
- establishing safety requirements for street vendors (Photo 7.7).

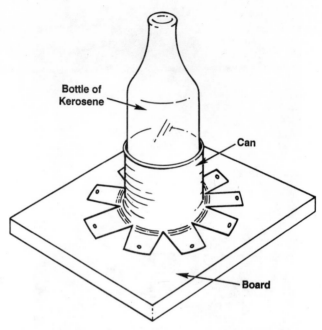

Figure 7.1: An inexpensive, more stable design for a kerosene bottle lamp. From Baker, S., Wintemute, G., The 'Ten Strategies' and Common Injury Problems. In, Principles for injury prevention in developing countries. WHO, Geneva, 1987, p. 24. Figure courtesy of Professor Susan Baker.

Examples of technologies that urgently need to be developed for LICs are:

- road designs which segregate traffic and also encourage motorists to drive at low speeds, popularly known as 'traffic-calming' measures.
- lightweight, comfortable, low-cost, and effective motorcycle crash helmets for tropical climates,
- simple-to-use screening tests for pesticide exposure, e.g., a finger-prick blood test for cholinesterase levels,
- inexpensive childproof containers for storing hazardous chemicals (gasoline, kerosene, pesticides, etc.) that non-literate adults can easily open (Photo 7.8).
- farming equipment with built in safety measures.

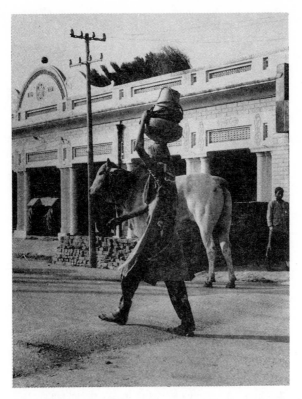

Photo 7.3: Non-vehicular traffic easily crosses this 'speed breaker' in a rural Indian village. Speed breakers are a low-cost environmental approach to reducing the speed of motorized vehicles in heavily-populated areas.

COMMUNITY INVOLVEMENT

People's potential for improving their own health and living conditions is enormous. The concept of community involvement for health has been seen as an antidote to health strategies that fail to encourage people to think and act for themselves, and that are often in conflict with the perceived priorities of local people. Furthermore, many important health promotion and curative activities such as injury prevention and first aid are only feasible as part of individual, family and community responsibilities.[10]

Many communities in LICs have local organizations that encourage

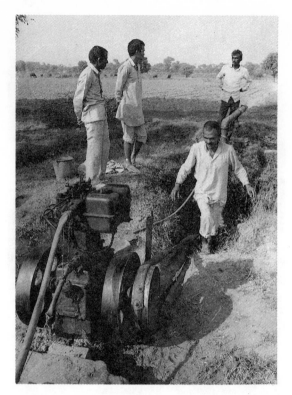

Photo 7.4: A long belt stretches from a diesel engine to a pump at the bottom of a ditch. Loose clothing can become entrapped between the belt and the drive shaft.

community involvement. Examples of such organizations are the 'Community Resilience Boards' in Indonesia which have a variety of sections, including health; local health committees in Pakistan that include mullahs, teachers and elders, and which provide a link between the health authorities and local communities; 'Community Action Boards' in Colombia; 'Quarter Councils' in the Sudan; and 'tabellas' in Somalia, whose unpaid members are chosen by the 50–100 families whom they represent.[11]

A major avenue for community participation in primary care programmes is the selection and training of community health workers (CHWs). CHWs provide preventive services aimed at individuals (e.g., education of parents on injury hazards), first aid, and follow-up

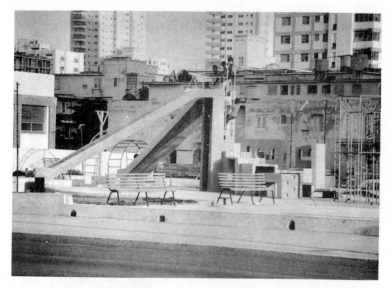

Photo 7.5: Despite its potential for falls, this children's slide in Havana is built over concrete. Grass or sand would offer a much more forgiving surface.

of injured or ill persons. They are often selected by the community to which they are accountable. CHWs are usually trained by the health teams at government health centres. The training often covers community organization, health care skills, such as first aid, and effective sharing of knowledge and skills. Their work is usually part-time and unpaid. Their knowledge of local customs, traditions, and culture, fluency with the language, and shared beliefs and experiences with the people they serve, make CHWs particularly effective in community-based health programmes.[5, 12]

EFFECTIVE COMMUNICATION

All community injury control programmes will have an educational component aimed at individuals, families, and entire neighborhoods or villages. Education involves the communication of ideas, knowledge, attitudes, and feelings. Efforts to communicate health messages may not be successful if only one or two communication channels

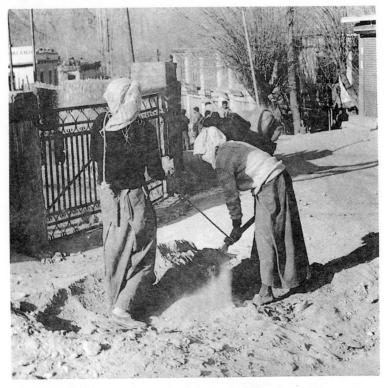

Photo 7.6: Orthopedic injuries are less likely when loads are lifted by more than one person. While doing road work in Ladakh, India, one woman holds the shovel handle while another helps lift with a rope attached near the top of blade.

are used, if people do not understand the messages they receive because of language difficulties or jargon, if the new knowledge conflicts with existing attitudes and beliefs, or if people do not have the financial or other resources to act on the information. UNICEF has outlined 'Twelve Steps in Health Communication' to promote child survival programmes.[13] The steps are equally applicable to community-based injury control efforts, or to any health education initiative:

1. Define clearly what health behaviour you are trying to promote. For example, cool water is the best first aid for burns,

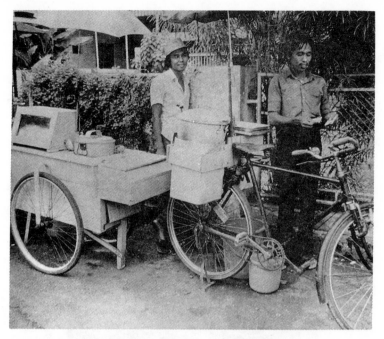

Photo 7.7: Both these vendors are selling hot soup (*baso*) in Jakarta. Children are sometimes burned when they dislodge the bicycle in the front; the cart in back is much more stable.

2. Decide exactly who in the population you are trying to influence,
3. Ask whether the new health behaviour requires new skills,
4. Learn about the present health knowledge, beliefs and behaviour of the target audience,
5. Enquire whether the health behaviour you are trying to promote has already been introduced to the community,
6. Investigate the target audience's present sources of information about health,
7. Select the communication channels and media which are most capable of reaching and influencing the target audience,
8. Design health messages which are easily understandable, culturally and socially appropriate, practical, brief, relevant, technically correct, and positive,
9. Develop and test your educational materials,

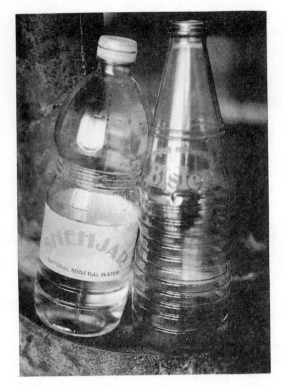

Photo 7.8: Both bottles are labelled, 'mineral water', but the one on the right contains kerosene for the stove. Unintentional kerosene poisonings are very common in LICs where child-proof containers are virtually unheard-of.

10. Synchronize your educational programme with other health and development services,
11. Evaluate whether the intended new behaviour is being carried out,
12. Repeat and adjust the messages at intervals over several years.

Both the mass media and interpersonal channels of communication can be powerful vehicles for health messages. In the past two decades, the number of radios in LICs has increased six-fold (to over 600 million), while the number of television sets has increased ten-fold (to almost 200 million). Over 8,000 newspapers are published throughout the world, nearly half in LICs.[13] Audience participation is possible

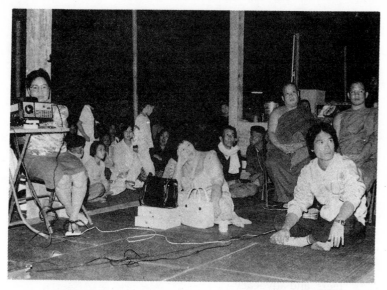

Photo 7.9: A Buddhist monastery in Chiang Mai, northern Thailand, becomes the site of a slide presentation on injury prevention. (Courtesy of Ajan Samboon, Chiang Mai.)

through the use of 'small media' namely video, films, slide shows, sound cassettes, and folk media, such as plays, puppet theatre, music and story-telling.

Many people in a community can be mobilized to become health communicators. Community health workers, medical professionals, and teachers are the most obvious candidates. Also to be considered are religious and spiritual leaders (Photo 7.9), trade union and co-operative leaders, employers and business leaders, government and community leaders, artists and entertainers, and leaders of women's organizations. However, all education initiatives must be a part of ongoing initiatives which improve services, designs of equipment and environment and law enforcement measures.[14]

FUNDING COMMUNITY-BASED INJURY PROGRAMMES

Funds are needed to plan, implement, evaluate, and maintain all types of health programmes. Yet in most LICs, health spending goes primarily to staff salaries, hospitals, and acute care.[5, 15] Even in HICs, monies available for prevention are limited when compared to expenditures on hospital care and out-patient treatment. A variety of funding sources must therefore be considered when seeking financial support for an innovative health programme. In high-income countries, funding sources include.[16]

- individuals (who, in the United States, contribute an estimated 80 per cent of all philanthropic gifts a year),
- foundations: non-profit organizations created by individuals or corporations to disburse grants for worthy efforts in their areas of interest,
- businesses and corporations: whose contributions can include cash grants, as well as human and material resources,
- government, at the local, regional, and national levels,
- religious institutions: from the local parish to national bodies, may offer financial support, meeting and office space, volunteers, and advocacy,
- community fund-raising organizations: non-profit organizations, such as United Way or the 'community chest,' consisting of groups of smaller organizations that pool their efforts in a fund-raising collection, usually with a common theme (women's issues, child health, the environment, etc.),
- community associations: many groups, such as service clubs (Lions, Elks, Shriners, Rotary) and professional groups (medical societies, teacher associations) engage in charitable activity as part of their reason for existence.

Health programmes in low-income countries may receive assistance from additional sources: international aid donors (e.g., Japan International Cooperation Agency, US Agency for International Development, Swedish International Development Authority), United Nations Organizations (UNICEF, UN Development Programme, UN Population Fund), regional banks and funds, and a number of international and national non-governmental organizations. Advice and assistance in finding donors can be obtained from local representatives of UNDP, WHO, or UNICEF. Guidelines for preparing a funding proposal are available from WHO (see also Learning Exercise 7, 'Writing a research proposal').[15, 17]

EXAMPLES OF COMMUNITY-BASED INJURY PREVENTION PROGRAMMES

Brazil's 'Alternative Services for Street Children' Project:[18-20]

In the early 1980's, estimates of the number of children 'living on the streets' in Brazil ranged from 7 to 20 million. The children were endangered by motor vehicles and other environmental hazards, as well as by exposure to prostitution, smuggling and drug traffic. They were often persecuted by police, exploited by adults, and threatened by peers. Many of these children were not entirely cut off from their families, but turned to the streets for their own subsistence or to supplement family income. They sought income as peddlers, waste-paper or rag pickers, shoe shiners, car washers, parking attendants, or pick-pockets.

Social assistance programmes, welfare facilities, and educational opportunities were scarce. The official system of institutional care was inadequate, inappropriate and too costly. Therefore, alternative approaches were sought by the Ministry of Social Welfare and Assistance, the National Child Welfare Foundation (FUNABEM), and UNICEF. An inventory of existing public and private projects for street children was undertaken, including regional meetings to explain different projects and discuss issues of mutual interest. A major strategy that arose from these meetings was to 'de-bureaucratize' the issue, to move it from the almost exclusive province of government professionals and technicians and open it to broad public influence and participation. This was because community programmes were observably more creative and competent in helping children, they had more practical ideas of what to do and how to do it, and they did it less expensively. Acting alone, the Government could not expect to reach even a small percentage of street children with its own resources, and it was unlikely to maintain the kind and quality of direct services needed in the face of political and administrative changes.

Local community groups and committees were set up in almost all major urban areas. Between 1982 and 1987, 480 training and review sessions were organized and programmes for street children rose from 22 to 370. The initial campaign spread to 25 states and territories. A Border Programme was designed for settlers' children in border districts. It provides training in agriculture, animal husbandry, electricity, carpentry, and other marketable skills to minors between 12 and 18 years old. A rural project, designed to reduce migration to urban centres and help rural youth acquire schooling and training, is carried out through 23 rural community development centres. The Non-Conventional Education programme develops alternative school policies, practices, and curricula to provide education for children deprived of access to formal education. The Project has published a series of technical pamphlets to focus attention on key issues: perceptions of street children, how to organize income-generating activities, adapting legislation to the special situation of street children, and establishing co-operative organizations.

There is still a tremendous gap between needs and services. It is estimated that 5,000 community programmes are necessary to effectively reach one million youngsters. The Alternative Services Project is a reminder that injury problems such as intentional, occupational, and pedestrian injuries involving street youths are sometimes best addressed from a broad-based, social context (work schemes, educational opportunities, etc.) rather than from a narrow health education or environmental approach.

Child Environment Advisors in South Australia

In South Australia, whose population is 1.25 million, over 500 deaths and 24,000 hospitalizations (11 per cent of the total) were injury-related in 1984. Children were an early target of injury prevention efforts. A community-based network of 'Child Environment Advisors' (CEA's) was established in 1981 to promote the involvement of parents in safety activities for children. The network differed from 'top-down' government programmes. It was designed to reach those sections of the community which had not been affected by existing educational efforts. An 'Accident Awareness Study' had shown that ethnic and low-income communities were unaware of preventive programmes and were not influenced by available brochures, media promotions, or poster campaigns.

The Child and Home Safety Centre in South Australia developed a programme based on the concept of community development. 'The belief that people with the real knowledge about the environment are those who live there, and that it is they who are in the best

position to influence their immediate surroundings.'[21] The programme recruited volunteers from the local community, whose
responsibility it was to assist parents in identifying and solving problems of home safety. To gain acceptance, the project was publicized
through local meetings, notice boards, ethnic churches, and personal
contacts with community leaders. Support was obtained from the
local community council which provided meeting facilities (Community Hall), publicity, and authority to make environmental changes
(such as repairing or replacing unsafe playground equipment).

Volunteers came from diverse cultural backgrounds and were
conversant with both the language and customs of the people in the
target communities (Greek, Spanish, Vietnamese, Lebanese, and
Australian). A series of workshops for volunteers provided them
with the factual material and interpersonal techniques to conduct
home visits and community safety surveys. The volunteers received
home safety check lists, poison charts, and numerous pamphlets
and posters in different languages to give to parents. The CEAs made
repeated visits to each household to develop personal relationships
with families.

The initial 3-month programme was evaluated using a questionnaire
survey.[22] Questionnaires were given to families visited by the CEAs
and to a comparison group of respondents randomly selected from
areas adjacent to the project communities. Families in the CEA group
were less likely to dress their children in loose pyjamas or a night-
dress (burn hazard), more likely to treat burns with cold water, and
more likely to provide appropriate first aid for falls. Recommendations for improved playground safety were submitted to the local
council. The positive results of the initial programme led to an extension of the community network approach to other council areas, and
a broadening of focus from injury prevention and emergency care to
overall preventive health. A Self-Help Health Care Manual was developed and translated into Greek, Italian, Polish, Serbo-Croatian,
Bulgarian, Spanish, Vietnamese, and Cambodian. The intent is to
establish health/environment networks for each ethnic community.

Village Wangkhoi: Injury Control and Primary Health Care

In 1985, The Nakhonsawan Research and Development Project
(NRDP) was established as a collaboration between the Ministry of

Public Health of Thailand, The ASEAN Training Centre for Primary Health Care Development, Mahidol University in Bangkok, and WHO. The major goals of the project were to develop appropriate models for assessing health needs and organizing health systems to optimize primary health care. The NRDP developed a system of education and training for health officers and workers, selection and recruitment of village health volunteers and communicators, activation of village committees, education and information for villagers, and technical support for village development projects.[23]

Nakhonsawan Province (NP) is 240 kilometres north of Bangkok, Thailand. It is divided into 12 amphoes (districts), 117 tambons (subdistricts), and 1,116 mubans (villages). The total population at the end of 1988 was 1.1 million people, 80 per cent of whom are farmers with an average per capita income of 13,167 baht ($526).

In 1986, health workers in the village of Wangkhoi requested technical assistance from the NRDP for village development projects, including injury prevention. A meeting was organized with village heads, project leaders, and local officials in Wangkhoi. Among the topics discussed were the concept of village development, village organizations and group representatives, and primary health care action programmes.

A village meeting was then held to promote local participation. At the meeting, villagers elected a committee with representatives from each of their residential clusters. They also elected 'health volunteers' to conduct a survey of illnesses and injuries in Wangkhoi and to help implement primary care activities. NRDP staff provided training to the volunteers and to the health post staff. The health volunteers learned how to collect illness and injury information on simple forms, which they completed during visits to village households.

Health volunteers, villagers, and local health workers met to discuss the survey results. The participants identified factors that contributed to individual health problems and they suggested possible solutions. They then prioritized problems according to the incidence and severity of each condition, treatment complexities, and individual interests and needs. Finally, a village plan of action was devised.

The villagers identified injuries as a leading cause of physical and financial losses. The major types of injuries were traffic crashes, falls, machinery, tools and sharp objects, and suicides and homicides. Wangkhoi village, where the main occupation is rice farming, had experienced rising injury rates from the use of farm machinery, fertilizers and pesticides, and motorized transportation. To address these problems, the health volunteers received training in the prevention and treatment. They disseminated this information through home visits, group discussions, village loud speakers, radio programmes, village meetings, and other media (leaflets, posters, booklets). Meetings were also held with government representatives (agriculture, drug and food control, police, schools) and private businesses involved in the production of farm machinery and chemicals. School children were taught about hazards to avoid during play, travel, and while working around the home. Student volunteers and scouts were trained to serve as traffic guards at crosswalks, and to recognize dangers in playgrounds, school yards, and at home. The police chief gave traffic safety sessions for villagers. Agricultural officials provided training on the safe handling of farm machines, transportation vehicles, and agricultural chemicals.

The community voluntary health services are currently operating through the support of the Village Fund Committee. The Village Fund is an innovative scheme that was introduced to insure the continuity of village programmes. Villagers contribute to the fund, each becoming a shareholding member. In addition to the shareholders contributions, the multi-purposes development fund receives funds from both government agencies and non-governmental organizations. Villagers borrow money for small-scale development projects (e.g., a fish hatchery, handicrafts centre, vegetable garden, or co-operative poultry scheme). A portion of the profits and interest are then returned to expand the Fund.

Community participation in Wangkhoi occurred through shared decision-making, direct labour, fund-raising, and maintenance of the primary care system. The principles of self-determination, self-reliance, and self-management were not mere concepts, but fundamental aspects of the injury control and primary health care programmes.[4, 24]

Applied Injury Prevention in Sweden: The Falkoping Experience

Injuries are the most common cause of death before the age of fifty in Sweden. Falls are the leading cause of injury-related mortality

(1,645 deaths), followed by traffic injuries (1,200 deaths). About 10 per cent of all hospital care is due to injuries.[25]

At the beginning of 1978, Sweden's Skaraborg County embarked on a community injury research project in conjunction with the Department of Social Medicine at the Karolinska Institute. The county's Community Health Unit began recording all injuries within the primary health area of Falkoping (population 32,000) and a control area, Lidkoping (34,000 inhabitants). Registration of injuries occurred through primary health care services (health centres, nursing homes, home medical services) and county and regional hospitals within the areas. (There are no private practitioners in the study areas.) Death certificates were also reviewed. The Community Health Care Unit was responsible for the distribution, collection and processing of the case report forms. Telephone surveys were carried out to obtain detailed information about occupational and home injuries. The registration system was continuous, covered all ages and all types of injuries, and operated as a routine in the course of regular work by nurses and doctors in the health centres and hospitals.

About 20 per cent of all acute visits were due to injuries. Of these, 25 per cent occurred at home and 20 per cent were occupational. Of the 18 fatal injuries in 1978, 10 occurred in homes, 5 in traffic, and 3 at unspecified locations.[26]

The intervention programme was begun in 1980. The programme was planned by a 'reference group' consisting of people from government (Community Health Unit, Social Welfare Office, Traffic Planning Office, Office of Recreation, etc.), community agencies (Tenant and Pensioner Associations, Farmers Health Care, Red Cross), the police, and other individuals (a local health planner and local politician, for example). For home injuries, children and the elderly were targeted as high-risk groups. Among occupational injuries, priority was given to falls, eye injuries, and crush injuries on farms and in industry.[27]

The intervention programme combined educational approaches and environmental changes in the home, at the workplace, and on public roads. Community education activities included exhibitions, posters, films, theatre performances, and evening presentations at schools, trade unions, and association meetings. A 3-day workplace safety programme was offered to industrial safety officers, work supervisors, safety engineers, occupational inspectors, and safety representatives in farming. Systematic safety visits were made to homes, schools, and day-nurseries with hazard checklists for children, the elderly, and farmers. In the traffic arena, eight road associations collaborated to identify high-risk locations for traffic injuries and to recommend improved construction, lighting, and crossing controls. Footpaths and cyclists, lanes were built where unprotected road-users (mainly school children) were at high risk of injury.

The results in Falkoping were dramatic: three years after the intervention began, the overall incidence of injuries declined by 30 per cent, from 113 injuries per 1,000 population per year, to 98 per 1,000. Home injuries were reduced by 27 per cent, traffic and occupational injuries by 28 per cent. Home injuries on farms decreased by almost 50 per cent. The incidence of occupational injuries among workers entitled to occupational health care decreased from 44.3 to 10.6 per 1,000 members per year. Injuries which were not subject to preventive measures did not change in incidence.[28] A special Public Health Board now has the responsibility for running the injury prevention programme. The programme mainly focuses on three areas: child safety education, road safety, and safety education for the elderly. The 30 per cent decrease in injury rate already achieved in 1981 has been maintained.[29]

COUNTERMEASURES FOR DRUNK DRIVING

The extent of world-wide alcohol consumption and the impact of alcohol-related crashes on motor vehicle injury rates are described in Chapter Four. In most HICs, public awareness of the risks of drunk driving and the possibility of severe legal penalties is high. Yet tens of thousands of people each year drink heavily and then drive their automobiles.[30]

Severe legal penalties can have a short-time effect. After passage of the British Road Safety Act in 1967, the per cent of fatally-injured drivers with blood alcohol levels above the legal limit fell sharply (Figure 7.2). However, once drivers recognized that their likelihood of arrest and penalty was extremely small, alcohol-involved crashes rose again.[31] The vast numbers of vehicles on the roads in HICs makes the probability of arrest low. Even when arrests are made, the judicial system has long delays and overcrowded jails that reduce the willingness of judges to impose severe penalties. Also, because drinking and driving is such a widespread social behavior in many HICs, judges, attorneys, and legislators are often reluctant to impose

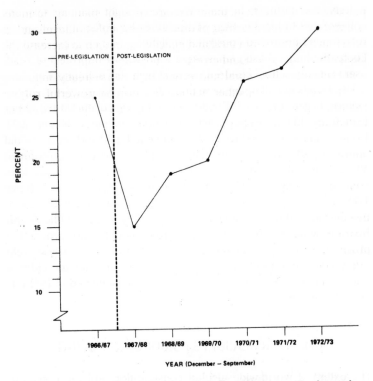

PRE-LEGISLATION | POST-LEGISLATION

PERCENT

YEAR (December – September)

Figure 7.2: The proportion of fatally-injured drivers with elevated blood alcohol concentrations fell after passage of the British Road Safety Act. However, it rose again steeply as motorists recognized that their risk of being arrested was small. From IIHS Status Report 1981; 16: 3. Insurance Institute for Highway Safety, Washington, D.C.

burdensome penalties such as prison terms to which they themselves may be subject. Severe penalties are even less likely to be imposed when the legal blood alcohol level is low. Many more drivers will be arrested if the legal limit is 0.04 per cent than if it is 0.08 per cent or 0.10 per cent.

An alternative to harsh penalties (such as mandatory prison terms) is the frequent imposition of less severe sanctions, such as fines, suspension of driving licenses, or confiscation of vehicles. Increasing the public's perception that a drunk driver is likely to get caught by the police and after the arrest, will likely experience consistently swift punishment is a strategy many nations are implementing. In many countries, random screening of drivers' breath alcohol levels at 'sobriety check-points' is a legal and effective approach to increase the likelihood of detection and arrest.

Because social, cultural and economic factors greatly influence alcohol consumption, other actions can have a powerful role in reducing drunk driving.[32, 33] The Surgeon-General of the United States, the country's leading public health official, recently called for increasing excise taxes on alcohol beverages, taxing beer, wine, and distilled spirits equally, based on alcohol content, and restricting advertising and marketing practices, especially those aimed at promoting alcoholic beverages among youth. Previously, raising the legal drinking age to 21 years greatly reduced the incidence of alcohol-related driving fatalities among young drivers.[34] In India's Maharashtra State, 'participatory research' led to massive community action to reduce alcohol consumption in 200 villages.[35] Villagers identified alcohol as a key community problem, recommended actions such as limiting the sale of alcohol, and mobilized widespread grassroots support.

REFERENCES

1. Manifesto for Safe Communities. First World Conference on Accident and Injury Prevention, Stockholm, September 17–20, 1989.
2. The National Committee for Injury Prevention and Control. 1989. Injury Prevention: Meeting the Challenge. Published by the Oxford University Press as a supplement to the *American Journal of Preventive Medicine* **5** (3).
3. Micik, S., Carlson, C. W. 1985. Preventing Childhood Injuries. North County Health Services, 348 Rancheros Drive, San Marcos, California 92069.
4. WHO 1989. Travelling Seminar on Formulating Guidelines for Safe Communities. Sweden-Thailand, September–October.
5. Morley, D., Lovel, H. 1986. My Name is Today. Macmillan Publishers, London.
6. Primary health care. 1978. Report of the International Conference on Primary Health Care, Alma-Ata, USSR, 6–12 September 1978. WHO, Geneva.
7. Evaluation of the strategy for health for all by the year 2000. Seventh report of the world health situation. Volume 1, Global review. WHO, Geneva, 1987.

8. Williams, G. 1988. WHO: reaching out to all. *World Health Forum* **9**: 185–99.
9. Proceedings of the Seminar on Accident and Injury Prevention Management at the Primary Health Care Level. Department of Medical Services, Ministry of Public Health, Bangkok, Thailand, 1987.
10. The Challenge of Implementation: District Health Systems for Primary Health Care. WHO, Geneva, 1988.
11. Tabibzadeh, I., Rossi-Espagnet, A., Maxwell, R. 1989. Spotlight on the cities: Improving urban health in developing countries. WHO, Geneva.
12. The Community Health Worker. WHO, Geneva, 1987.
13. All for Health: A resource book for Facts for Life. UNICEF, New York, 1990.
14. Marketing of Traffic Safety. OECD, Paris, 1993.
15. Dowling, M. A. C. 1989. Raising funds for health programmes. WHO, Geneva. HMD/89.4.
16. Seltzer, M. 1987. Securing Your Organization's Future. The Foundation Center, New York.
17. Janovsky, K. 1987. Project formulation and proposal writing. WHO, Geneva. WHO/EDUC/87.187.
18. Projeto Alternativas de Atendimento aos Meninos de Rua (Alternative services for Street Children Project). 1988. In: 'The emerging response to child labour.' Conditions of Work Digest, ILO, Geneva, **7**: 97–101.
19. Myers, W. 1988. Alternative services for street children: The Brazilian approach. In: Bequele, A., Boyden, J. (eds), Combating child labour. ILO, Geneva.
20. Michaels, J. 1990. Brazil launches program to help needy children. *Christian Science Monitor*, June 4, p. 4.
21. Whitelaw, S. 1991. Evaluation of educational projects in Australia. In: Manciaux, M., Romer, C. J., Accidents in Childhood and Adolescence: The Role of Research. WHO, Geneva, chapter 14, pp. 161–72.
22. Depold, R. P., Steidl, P. E., Whitelaw, S. 1983. Development and evaluation of a community self-help programme: the network of child-environment advisors. National Safety Council of Australia, Bowden, S.A.
23. Svetsreni, T. 1989. Nakhonsawan PHC support research and development process toward community self-managed accident prevention model. Paper prepared for the Sweden-Thailand Traveling Seminar on Models for Accident Prevention in Local Communities. September.
24. Havanonda, S., Svestsreni, T., Bhokakul, P. 1987. Village Wangkhoi: A case of PHC in accident and injuries prevention. In: Proceedings of the Seminar on Accident and Injury Prevention Management at the Primary Health Care Level. Pattaya, Thailand, 3–5 March 1987. Department of Medical Services, Ministry of Public Health, Bangkok.
25. Schelp, L., Svanstrom, L. 1986. One-year incidence of home accidents in a rural Swedish municipality. *Scand J Soc Med* **14**: 75–82.

26. Schelp, L. 1984. Accident prevention within a primary health area. In: Berfenstam, R., Kohler, L. (eds), Methods and Experience in Planning for Accident Prevention. The Nordic School of Public Health, Stockholm, pp. 173-7.
27. Schelp, L., Svanstrom, L. 1986. One-year incidence of occupational accidents in a rural Swedish municipality. *Scand J Soc Med* **14**: 197–204.
28. Schelp, L., Svanstrom, L. 1989. Outcome of a community intervention program on unintentional injuries. Paper presented at the First World Conference on Accident and Injury Prevention, September 17–20, Stockholm, Sweden.
29. Research on Community Safety Promotion. Karolinska Institute, Department of Social Medicine, Kronan Health Centre, Sundbyberg, Sweden, 1989.
30. Ross, H. L. 1981. Deterring the Drinking Driver. Lexington Books, Lexington.
31. Drinking-Driving Laws. Insurance Institute for Highway Safety Status Report 1981. **16**: 1–5.
32. Problems related to alcohol consumption. Report of a WHO Expert Committee. Technical Report Series 650, WHO, Geneva, 1980.
33. Factors potentially associated with reductions in alcohol-related traffic fatalities—United States, 1990 and 1991. *Morbidity and Mortality Weekly Reports* 1992. **41** (48): 893–9.
34. Surgeon General's Workshop on Drunk Driving Proceedings, 1989. US Public Health Service, Office of the Surgeon-General, 5600 Fishers Lane, Rockville, MD 20857 USA.
35. Bang, A. T., Bang, R. A. 1991. Community participation in research and action against alcoholism. *World Health Forum* **12**: 104–9.

FURTHER READINGS

1. Accident and injury prevention at the primary health care level. WHO Injury Prevention Programme, Geneva, 1987.
2. Moore, J. D., Gerken, E. A. (eds), You can make a difference: Preventing injuries in your community. Available from the UNC Injury Prevention Center, 310 Carrington Hall, University of North Carolina, Chapel Hill, NC 27599-7460.
3. Community Health Surveys: A Practical Guide for Health Workers. 6 Volumes, 1981–9. International Epidemiological Association. Available from WHO Regional Offices.
4. Criteria for the development of health promotion and education programmes. *American Journal of Public Health* 1987. **77**: 89–92.
5. Raymond. J. S., Pastrick, W. 1988. Empowerment for primary health care

and child survival: Escalating community participation, community competence, and self-reliance in the Pacific. *Asia-Pacific Journal of Public Health* **2**: 90–5.

6. Amonoo-Lartson, R., Ebrahim, G., Lovel, H. J., Ranken, J. P. 1984. District Health Care. Macmillan Press, London.

7. Education for Health. A newsletter from the Division of Health Education and Health Promotion, WHO, Geneva.

8. A tale of two cities: Strategies for DWI deterrence. Insurance Institute for Highway Safety Status Report 1988; 23: 1–2.

9. Christoffel, T. 1984. Using roadblocks to reduce drunk driving: Public health or law and order? *American Journal of Public Health* **74**: 1028–30.

10. Alcohol Policies. WHO Regional Publications, European Series No. 18. Regional Office for Europe, WHO, Copenhagen, 1985.

11. Drug dependence and alcohol-related problems: A manual for community health workers with guidelines for trainers. WHO, Geneva, 1986.

12. The influence of alcohol and drugs on driving. EURO Reports and Studies, No. 38, 1981.

13. Drugs, Driving and Traffic Safety. WHO Offset Publication No. 78, 1983.

14. *OECD* road safety research: a synthesis. OECD, Paris, 1986.

15. Mohan, D. 1992. Vulnerable Road Users: An era of neglect. *Journal of Traffic Medicine* **20**: 121–8.

Afterword

One of the most exciting aspects about the field of injury control is that it is ever expanding. Today, all forms of injury—motor vehicle crashes, burns, falls, drownings, poisonings, suicides, homicides, child abuse are proper subjects of scholarly investigation and public health action.[1-5] New injury problems which require original research and fresh solutions appear almost daily: burns in tanning salons, falls from skateboards, hearing loss from rock music concerts, radiation from computer display terminals, deaths from automatic garage doors, drownings in hot tubs, newly-formulated industrial chemicals (500 to 1,000 are introduced each year to the 70,000 presently in everyday use),[6] and even new types of motorized vehicles. For example, all-terrain vehicles (ATV's) were virtually unknown in the United States in the 1970's, but became a wildly popular and very injurious means of 'entertainment' for young people in the next decade.

Sales of ATV's increased from 136,000 in 1980 to 484,000 in 1983. An estimated 1.25 million were in use by 1984. Of the more than 27,000 ATV-associated injuries treated in emergency rooms during 1982 to 1983, 11 per cent required hospitalization and at least 15 deaths occurred. Nearly one-half of the victims are under 18 years of age. The sudden appearance of ATV injuries seems to parallel the increased advertising that these vehicles are receiving both locally and nationally.[7]

For many types of injuries such as motor vehicle crashes, firearm deaths, flame and scald burns drastic reductions in morbidity and mortality are achievable with current information and technology.[8, 9] These areas require a shift from research to activism, finding ways to implement countermeasures of proven effectiveness in the community in the face of economic, social, and political barriers.[10-12] The field of injury control is also expanding (Figure 8.1). Injury control researchers are paying more attention to topics such as

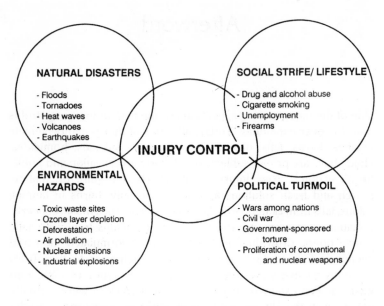

Figure 8.1: The field of injury control is expanding.

environmental hazards (over 50 million metric tons of toxic wastes are produced yearly in the U.S. alone),[6] natural disasters, political turmoil, military actions, and the threat of nuclear war.[13-24] The tools of injury control research namely epidemiology, Haddon's matrix, the '4 Es' are applicable to these areas as well.

New research and new injury prevention advocates will be needed to meet the continuing challenge posed by injuries throughout the world. We look forward to learning about the successes of our readers in making this world a safer place to live in.

REFERENCES

1. Accident Prevention: Global Medium-Term Programme, 1990-5. WHO Injury Prevention Programme, Geneva, 1988. APR/MTP/88.1.
2. Romer, C. J. 1993. Injury and violence: from fate to health. Inter-regional

Seminar on Methods for Community Safety Programme Planning. World Health Organization, Geneva.

3. Committee on Trauma Research, National Research Council: Injury in America. National Academy Press, Washington, D.C., 1985.

4. Violence and the Public's Health. *Health Affairs* 1993. **12** (4): 1–262.

5. Violence—A Matter of Health. *World Health Magazine*, January–February 1993, WHO, Geneva.

6. Postel, S. 1988. Controlling toxic chemicals. In: State of the World 1988. Worldwatch Institute, New York, p. 119.

7. Sneed, R. C., Stover, S. L., Fine, P. R. 1986. Spinal cord injury associated with all-terrain vehicle accidents. *Pediatrics* **77**: 271–4.

8. The National Committee for Injury Prevention and Control: Injury Prevention: Meeting the Challenge. Published by Oxford University Press as a supplement to the *American Journal of Preventive Medicine* **5** (3), 1989.

9. Rivara, F. P. 1985. Traumatic deaths of children in the United States: Currently available prevention strategies. *Pediatrics* **75**: 456–62.

10. Wilson, M. H., Baker, S. P., Teret, S. P. et al. 1991. Saving Children: A Guide to Injury Prevention. Oxford University Press, New York.

11. Creating Caring Communities: Blueprint for an effective federal policy on child abuse and neglect. US Advisory Committee on Child Abuse and Neglect, September 15, 1991.

12. Handle Life With Care: Prevent Violence and Negligence. Information Kit, World Health Day, 7 April 1993. Injury Prevention Programme, World Health Organization, Geneva, 1993.

13. Coping with natural disasters: The role of local health personnel and the community. WHO, Geneva, 1989.

14. Duclos, P., Isaacson, J. 1987. Preventable deaths related to floods. *American Journal of Public Health* **77**: 1474.

15. Bernstein, R. S., Baxter, P. J., Buist, A. S. 1986. Introduction to the epidemiologic aspects of explosive volcanism. *American Journal of Public Health* (Supplement); **76**: 3–9.

16. A System for Prevention, Assessment, and Control of Exposures and Health Effects from Hazardous Sites. Centers for Disease Control, Atlanta, 1984.

17. Roth, E. F., Lunde, I., Boysen, G. et al. 1987. Torture and its treatment. *American Journal of Public Health* **77**: 1404–6.

18. Nicaragua Health Study Collaborative. 1989. Health effects of the war in two rural communities in Nicaragua. *American Journal of Public Health* **79**: 424–9.

19. Yach, D. 1988. The impact of political violence on health and health services in Cape Town, South Africa, 1986: Methodological problems and preliminary results. *American Journal of Public Health* **78**: 772–6.

20. Nightingale, E. O., Hannibal, K., Gieger, J. et al. 1990. Apartheid medicine: Health and human rights in South Africa. *Journal of the American Medical Association* **264** (16): 1097–2102.
21. Principles of studies on diseases of suspected chemical etiology and their prevention. Environmental Health Criteria No. 72. WHO, Geneva, 1987.
22. Guidelines on studies in environmental epidemiology. International Programme on Chemical Safety. Environmental Health Criteria 27, WHO, Geneva, 1983.
23. Effects of nuclear war on health and health services. WHO, Geneva, 1987.
24. Nuclear power: Accidental releases—Practical guidance for public health action. WHO Regional Publications, European Series, No. 21, WHO, Copenhagen, 1987.

Appendix A

SELECTED KEY REFERENCES IN INJURY CONTROL

1   Accident Facts. 1994. National Safety Council, Itasca, IL, 1994.
2. Baker, S. P., O'Neill, B., Ginsburg, M., Li, G. 1992. *The Injury Fact Book* (Second Edition) Oxford University Press, New York.
3. Barss, P., Smith, G. S., Mohan, D., Baker, S. P. 1991. Injuries to adults in developing countries: Epidemiology and policy. The World Bank, Washington, D.C.
4. Graitcer, P. L. 1992. Injury surveillance in developing countries. MMWR–CDC Surveillance Suymmaries, 41 (SS-1): 15–20.
5. Korbin, J. E. (ed.). 1981. Child Abuse and Neglect: Cross-Cultural Perspectives. University of California Press, Berkeley.
6. Levinson, D. 1989. Family Violence in Cross-Cultural Perspective. Sage Publications, Newbury Park.
7. Manciaux, M., Romer, C. J. (eds). 1991. Accidents in Childhood and Adolescence: The Role of Research. World Health Organization, Geneva.
8. Mohan, D. (ed.). 1991. The Vulnerable Road User: International Conference on Traffic Safety. MacMillan India, Delhi.
9. Mohan, D. 1984. Accidental death and disability in India: A stock-taking. *Accident Analysis and Prevention* 16: 279–88.
10. National Committee for Injury Prevention and Control: Injury Prevention: Meeting the Challenge. *American Journal of Preventive Medicine* Supplement, Oxford University Press, 1989.
11. Rice, D. P., MacKenzie, E. J. and Associates. 1989. The Cost of Injury in the United States. San Francisco CA: Institute for Health and Aging, University of California and Injury Prevention Center, The John Hopkins University.
12. Robertson, L. S. 1992. *Injury Epidemiology*. Oxford University Press, New York.
13. Romer, C. J. 1993. Injury and violence: From fate to health. Inter-regional seminar on methods for community safety

programme planning. Injury Prevention Programme, WHO, Geneva.

14. Rosenberg, M. L., Fenley, M. A. 1991. Violence in America. National Academy Press, Washington, D.C.

15. Smith, G. S., Barss, P. 1991. Unintentional injuries in developing countries. The epidemiology of a neglected problem. *Epidemiologic Reviews* **13**: 228–66.

16. Stansfield, S. K., Smith, G. S., McGreevey, W. P. 1990. Injury and poisoning. In: Jamison, D. T., Mosley, W. H., The World Bank Health Sector Priorities Review. The World Bank, Washington, D.C., Chapter 24.

17. Trinca, G. W., Johnston, I. R., Campbell, B. J. et al. 1988. Reducing Traffic Injury: A Global Challenge. Royal Australasian College of Surgeons, Melbourne.

18. Wilson, M. H., Baker, S. P., Teret, S. P., Shock, S., Garbarino, J. 1991. *Saving Children*. Oxford University Press, New York.

19. World Development Report 1993: Investing in Health. Oxford University Press, New York, 1993.

20. World Health Day 1993, Information Kit: Handle life with care: Prevent violence and negligence. WHO, Geneva, 7 April 1993.

Appendix B

INJURY CONTROL ORGANIZATIONS AND AGENCIES

American Academy of Pediatrics Committee on Accident and Poison Prevention

141 Northwest Point Blvd.
P.O. Box 927
Elk Grove Village, IL 60009–0927

The COAPP issues policy statements and recommendations on injury problems related to children. Its Accident Prevention Newsletter is published two times a year to provide current information on pediatric injury control including abstracts of recent articles and reports of product hazards.

American Association for Automotive Medicine (AAAM)

c/o Dr Ted Tong
Arizona Poison and Drug Information Center
Health Sciences Center, Room 3204 K
1502 N Campbell
Tucson, AZ 85725

AAAM publishes a Quarterly Journal, Proceedings of its annual meetings, and revisions of the Abbreviated Injury Scale.

American Association of Poison Control Centers

2025 I Street, N.W.
Suite 105
Washington, D.C. 20006

Since 1958, the AAPCC has worked with poison centers, government and industry to improve the treatment of poisonings asnd prevent accidental poisonings. It provides members services to facilitate education, research and comprehensive poison treatment information.

Centers for Disease Control (CDC)

Atlanta, Georgia 30333

CDC is best known for its work on infectious diseases. However, the public health and epidemiologic resources of CDC also are applied to injury control through its National Center for Injury Prevention and Control, Center for Health Promotion and Education, Emergency Response Coordination Group, Division of Environmental Hazards and Health Effects, and National Institute for Occupational Safety and Health.

Education Development Center, Inc.

55 Chapel Street, Newton, MA 02160 USA

Provides technical assistance to health agencies and academic programs seeking to develop injury prevention programmes.

European Consumer Product Safety Association (ECPSA)

P.O. Box 5169
1007 AD Amsterdam, The Netherlands

ECPSA has secretariats of public relations and education, research and documentation, and product safety. It conducts conferences and seminars for professional training, coordinates research activities and monitors projects dealing with home and leisure accidents. ECPSA organizes international campaigns for safer products and maintains a specialized library and information network of safety experts and consumer product safety activities.

Insurance Institute for Highway Safety (IIHS)

1005 North Glebe Road, Suite 800
Arlington, VA 22201 USA

IIHS analyzes insurance claims data and conducts research (biomechanical, epidemiologic, engineering) in all aspects of motor vehicle injury reduction. The Institute has created superb films on topics such as air bags, highway hazards, and child passenger safety.

It issues a *Status Report* containing news and research results on highway safety.

Inter-American Safety Council

33 Park Place
Englewood, New Jersey 07631 USA

IASC offers publications, technical consultations, and statistical services, sponsors safety awards programmes, conferences, and courses; and provides a safety instructor certification programme. Its biennial catalogue lists safety posters, films, slides, books, and other educational materials.

International Association for Accident and Traffic Medicine (IAATM)

Postfack 1644
5751 46 Uppsala
Sweden

Members of IAATM are physicians and scientists from 43 countries. Through its Journal of Traffic Medicine and at its meetings, IAATM disseminates scientific information on traffic medicine, including alcohol-related problems, in road, rail, air and sea transport.

International Association of Agricultural Medicine and Rural Health (IAAMRH)

Saku Central Hospital
197, Usuda
Minamisaku-gun, Nagano 384–03
Japan

Publishes a quarterly journal and conducts regional symposia on all aspects of health in the agricultural sector.

International Commission for the Prevention of Alcoholism and Drug Dependency

12501 Old Columbia Pike
Silver Spring, MD 20904 USA

Members represent 120 countries with national committees in over

50 countries. Conducts seminars, consultations, world congresses, facilitates establishment of national comittees.

International Council on Alcohol and Addictions (ICAA)

Case postale 189
1001 Lausanne
Switzerland

ICAA maintains an international reference library, organizes conferences and training courses on alcohol, tobacco, and other drug dependence problems.

International Electrotechnical Commission (IEC)

3, rue de Varembe
Case postale 131
1211 Geneva 20
Switzerland

The IEC prepares technical reports and issues standards in the fields of electricity and electronics.

International Ergonomics Association (IEA)

Central Advisory Group on Ergonomics
Netherlands Railways
NL-3511 Utrecht
Netherlands

With Federated Societies in 20 countries, IEA conducts research on topics such as office automation, work design, and ergonomics in developing countries. It also holds conferences and symposia and publishes a quarterly journal, *Ergonomics.*

International Federation for Housing and Planning (IFHP)

Wassenaarseweg 43
NL-2596 CG Den Haag
Netherlands

IFHP has standing committees on housing, traffic problems, urban renewal and land policy. It organizes international seminars, training courses, and study tours.

International Federation of Chemical, Energy and General Workers' Unions (ICEF)

109, Av. Emile de Beco
B-1050 Brussels
Belgium

ICEF has over six million members in 200 affiliated trade unions in 72 countries. The organization collects information on worker's issues, including health, ergonomics and safety, conducts research, provides assistance for training programmes, especially in developing countries; and collaborates in standard setting to reduce occupational risks.

International Federation of Pedestrians (IFP)

3500 Race Street
Philadelphia, PA 19104-2440
USA

IFP unites national associations for protection of pedestrian's rights and safety. IFP issues a quarterly newsletter and sponsors congresses and educational programmes of interest to pedestrians.

International Federation on Ageing (IFA)

601 East Street NW
Washington, D.C. 20049-1170
USA

IFA has a membership from 95 national associations in 46 countries. It conducts symposia, conferences, and skills exhange programmes on all aspects of the well being of elderly people throughout the world.

International Foundation for Road Safety in Developing Countries

c/o PRI
75, rue de Mamer
L-8081 Bertrange
Luxembourg

Founded in 1983 by the International Road Safety Organisation,

IFRSDC encourages the creation and expansion of road safety associations in developing countries.

International Occupational Safety and Health Information Centre Bit – CIS

4, rue de Morillons
CH 1211 Geneva 22
Switzerland

CIS operates within the International Labour Organization (ILO), a specialized agency of the United Nations. CIS reviews global occupational safety and health literature in areas such as industrial hygiene, occupational medicine, toxicology, injury prevention, safety engineering, ergonomics and stress. CIS abstracts are published in a computer produced periodical. Information sheets offer practical guides on safety and health subjects for the shop floor level. Bibliographic searches are available on-line or on request.

International Organization of Consumers Unions

Emmastraat 9
NL-2595 EG The Hague
Netherlands

A non-profit foundation which supports its member consumer organizations from 51 countries, promotes the expansion of the consumer movement worldwide, and functions as an international consumer advocate at the United Nations and in other fora. It publishes newsletters, consumer handbooks, and other materials. The IOCU maintains a specialized library with legislative, technical and educational information relevant to consumer interests, and supports studies on the sale of dangerous drugs and pesticides in Third World countries.

International Organization for Standardization (ISO)

1, rue de Varembe
Case postale 56
CH-1211 Geneva 20
Switzerland

ISO publishes the KWIC (Key-Word-in-Context) Index of international standards. Together with the International Electrotechnical Commission (IEC), ISO has published more than 8,000 international standards ranging from maximum limits for pesticide residues and techniques for determining the maximum speed of motorcyles to criteria for seat belt anchorages on agricultural tractors. KWIC is updated every two years.

International Paediatric Association (IPA)

Chateau de Longchamp
Bois de Boulogne
F-75016 Paris
France

IPA conducts regional and international seminars and symposia on topics such as accidents in childhood, adolescent health, child abuse, and preventable handicaps. IPA member organizations have collaborated with WHO in an international study of childhood injuries.

International Physicians for the Prevention of Nuclear War (IPPNW)

126 Rogers Street
Cambridge,
Massachusetts 02142
USA

IPPNW was founded in 1980 as a result of a meeting between American and Soviet physicians. It has members from 55 countries who apply their medical expertise to the problem of preventing nuclear war and controlling the nuclear arms race. IPPNW designs curricula on aspects of nuclear war for medical schools, conducts special projects (such as on the psychological effects of the arms race on children), and provides information to the public through lay and medical publications.

International Radiation Protection Association (IRPA)

Postbus 662
NL-5600 AR Eindhoven
Netherlands

Encourages the establishment of radiation protection societies and standards throughout the world, promotes scientific meetings and research in radiation protection.

International Research Council on Biokinetics of Impacts (IRCOBI)

109 Avenue
Salvador Allende,
69500 Bron,
France.

IRCOBI was founded in 1971 by a group of European Researchers with the aims of advancing the study of biomechanics of impact trauma. IRCOBI organises an annual meeting with international participation.

International Road Safety Organization

75 rue de Mamer
L-8081 Bertrange
Luxembourg

IRSO studies road safety problems in conjunction with its member organizations from 57 countries. Its quarterly publication appears in English, French and German. IRSO also sponsors international congresses and competitions (e.g., a television film competition on road safety).

International Society for Burn Injuries (ISBI)

c/o Dr J.A. Boswick
2005 Franklin Street
Building 1, Suite 660
Denver, Colorado 80205
USA

ISBI promotes research in the clinical, social, and preventive aspects of burns. Encourages improved burn care through congresses, symposia, and providing visiting lectures.

International Society for the Prevention of Child Abuse and Neglect (ISPCAN)

1205 Oneida Street
Denver, CO 80220
USA

ISPCAN was founded as a society to work for the prevention of child abuse and neglect by facilitating the sharing of knowledge and experience. ISPCAN publishes a newsletter and journal, and sponsors international conferences. Topics of interest to ISPCAN members include street children, armed conflict and political violence, sexual exploitation of children, networking of concerned professionals and volunteers, and community-based activities to prevent child abuse and neglect.

International Union for Health Education

Institute Sante et Development
15–21, rue de l'Ecole de Medecine
F-75270 Paris Cedex 06
France

Facilitates international exchange of information and experiences, and promotes scientific research in the field of health education.

National Highway Traffic Safety Administration

400 Seventh Street S.W. (NTS-11)
Washington, D.C. 20590
USA

Provides technical and financial assistance to state and local governments and works with private organizations to promote safety programs. Offers brochures, fact sheets, and research publications.

National Safe Kids Campaign

111 Michigan Avenue NW
Washington, D.C. 20010–2970
USA

Promotes child safety through state and local committees, legislative action, and publication of informational materials.

National Safety Council (NSC)

1121 Spring Lake Drive
Itasca, Illinois 60143
USA

A non-governmental public service organization that provides safety services and information to industry, insurance companies, safety organizations, government departments, schools and individuals. NSC publishes a yearly summary of national injury statistics titled, *Accident Facts*.

Trauma Foundation

Building One, Room 400
San Francisco General Hospital
San Francisco, CA 94110

A non-profit, membership supported foundation that publishes the Injury Prevention Network Newsletter. The newsletter discusses current research, strategies and actions to prevent injuries.

US Consumer Product Safety Commission

Washington, D.C. 20207
USA

The CPSC has broad authority to issue and enforce safety standards governing the design, construction, contents, performance, packaging and labelling of over 10,000 consumer products. Its National Electronic Injury Surveillance System (NEISS) monitors a sample of hospital emergency rooms for consumer product injuries. CPSC also conducts studies, tests products, and publishes educational materials for consumers.

World Federation of Public Health Associations (WFPHA)

c/o American Public Health Association
1015 Fifteenth Street, N.W.
Washington, D.C. 20005
USA

WFPHA holds annual meetings in Geneva during the World Health Assembly and international congresses every three years. It sponsors special studies and projects, and publishes monographs and reports, on public health topics of international significance.

Appendix C

COMPUTERIZED INFORMATION SYSTEMS

Computerized information systems play an increasing role in patient care, teaching, and research in all aspects of health, including injury control. The Medical Literature Access Retrieval Service (MEDLARS) has numerous databases that can be accessed in a variety of ways from countries all over the world: directly via modem, through 'GRATEFUL MED' (described below), or through Internet (a global information network). Medlars is also available on CD-ROM. GRATEFUL MED is a user-friendly system. It is a software package on a floppy disk that allows users to use their personal computers to search the data files: MEDLINE, CATLINE, DIRLINE, and TOXLINE, among others. MEDLINE and its backfiles contain more than 5 million references to journal articles from 1966 to the present. It is the major source for worldwide medical literature with articles from over 3800 of the world's journals. CATLINE contains 600,000 records for books and serials. GRATEFUL MED may be run on an IBM PC, IBM-compatible, or MacIntosh computer equipped with a modem.

Another computerized database maintained by NLM is called DIRLINE: Directory of Information Resources on Line. It contains information about over 15,000 public and private organizations (primarily health and biomedical) considered to be resource centers because of their willingness to respond to public inquiries in their areas of specialty. (For further information on GRATEFUL MED and DIRLINE, contact: MEDLARS Management Section, National Library of Medicine, 8600 Rockville Pike, Bethesda, Maryland 20894 USA; or INTERNET mms@nlm.nih.gov).

EMBASE is a service of Excerpta Medica and provides abstracts of biomedical articles from 3,500 journals around the world. Like MEDLINE, EMBASE covers a broad range of biomedical and public health topics, including drug and pharmaceutical literature, environmental health, pollution, and forensic science. It is available from a variety of data-base vendors. (Information: Elsevier Scientific Publishers, North America Database Department, 52 Vanderbilt Avenue, New York, NY 10017 USA, or Elsevier Scientific Publishers, Molenwerf-1, 1014 AG Amsterdam, the Netherlands.)

The CDC's Centre for Health Promotion and Education produces a computerized list called the 'Health Education subfile of the Combined Health Information Database.' The subfile includes articles, monographs, proceedings, reports, curricular materials, unpublished documents and program descriptions relating to patient education, school and community health education, occupational health and risk-reduction education, and professional training (Further information: Combined Health Information Database, 23114 East Jefferson Street, Suite 401, Rockville, MD 20852, USA).

Systems with important clinical applications, which also can be very valuable for injury control research, include the following:

Poisindex is a toxicology information system 'designed to identify and provide ingredient information on commercial, industrial, pharmaceutical and botanical substances.' It also provides treatment/management protocols if substances are ingested, absorbed, or inhaled. Over 410,000 substances are included indexed by brand/trade name, generic/chemical name, common names and common misspellings. Each treatment/management protocol includes a description of clinical effects, pharmacology, treatment, range of toxicity, and references. A botanical and zoological section has plant descriptions with identification of toxic chemicals, treatment protocols and photographs of poisonous plants, mushrooms, and snakes. The system is available by microfiche, laser disc for use with personal computers, and computer tapes for mainframe applications.

Drugdex provides information on drug dosages, pharmacokinetics, adverse reactions, drug interactions, clinical applications, contraindications, precautions, effects in pregnancy, and patient instructions. It covers both prescription and over-the-counter drugs available in the United States as well as non-US preparations.

Emergindex is an acute care information system with clinical reviews of subjects, clinical abstracts of the world's medical literature for use in continuing education and research, detailed lists of etiologies for specific patient complaints, and a computerized topic search in emergency and critical care medicine. (For further information on Poisondex, Drugdex, and Emergindex: Micromedex Inc., 600 Grant Street, Denver, Colorado 80203-3527.)

Toxline covers the adverse effects of chemicals, drugs, and physical agents on living systems. Approximately 120,000 citations are added to the database each year.

Appendix D

LEARNING EXERCISES

EXERCISE 1:
INTERPRETING DATA FROM MEDICAL RECORDS*

The rate of hospitalization of children with injuries in one community (called Sadcom) was three times that of the surrounding region (called Onestate). To determine the reasons, researchers analyzed mortality and hospitalization data, and performed an in-depth review of medical records.

A. What are possible reasons for such a large difference in hospitalization rates for injuries in the two populations. Consider statistical factors as well as factors related to the host, agent, and environment.

B. What additional information and calculations would you need to decide which of the possible factors are unlikely and which might actually account for the higher injury rate among children in Sadcom?

ANSWERS

A. Among the Possible Explanations
for the High Injury Rate are:

1. An artefact of reporting:
   a. Sadcom hospitals have more complete reporting of injuries, either because their medical records are better, or

---

* This exercise was adapted from material contained in Berger LR and Kitzes J: Injuries to children in a Native American community. *Pediatrics* July, 1989.)

because residents of Onestate are more likely to use hospitals outside of their immediate community.

b. Sadcom hospitals define a broader range of conditions as 'injuries' (e.g., including intentional injuries, poisonings, etc.).

c. 'Children' are defined differently in the two reporting systems: In Sadcom, up to 18 years of age while in Onestate, up to 14 years. This would obviously produce a higher numerator for Sadcom.

2. Uncertain denominator data: The population of Sadcom children is underestimated, leading to higher calculated rates of injury, or the population of Onestate is overestimated, producing artificially lower rates.

3. Lack of age-adjustment: If Sadcom has many young infants compared to Onestate, and the rate of injury to infants is higher than for older children, the rate for the overall child population in Sadcom will be higher.

4. Lower socio-economic status of Sadcom: There is a strong association between poverty and many types of injury.

5. Different thresholds for hospitalization: Doctors in Sadcom may be more likely to hospitalize children for minor injuries that are treated and released in other Onestate hospitals. For example, some physicians routinely hospitalize children with any form of head trauma, others often let the children be observed at home by the parents.

6. An increase in a specific type of injury. Sadcom may have a busy highway running down the center of town, dividing homes on one side of the road from schools and playgrounds on the other.

7. Psychosocial/lifestyle factors: Parental supervision may be less in Sadcom because of high rates of alcoholism or drug abuse or family violence may be more prevalent resulting in high rates of child abuse.

B. Ways to Decide Among the Above Possibilities Include:

1. Artefacts of reporting: review the reporting systems of hospitals in each community by visiting the medical records departments, conduct a utilization study to determine what percent

of hospitalizations are 'captured' by the reporting hospitals in each population.

2. Denominator data: Determine if the population estimates were determined by the same techniques, conduct a sensitivity analysis with different denominators for each community to see if the discrepancy in rates could be largely accounted for by uncertainty in the denominator.

3. Lack of age-adjustment: Determine the age distribution of each community, if there are large differences, calculate age-specific rates of hospitalization.

4. Lower socio-economic status: Obtain economic data from each community regarding income distribution and unemployment rates.

5. Different thresholds of hospitalization: Examine rates of outpatient visits for injuries. If the ratio of rates for injury-related outpatient visits between Sadcom and Onestate is the same as the ratio of hospitalization rates, then the higher hospitalization rates in Sadcom do reflect increased injury rates in the community and not a lower threshold for hospitalization by Sadcom physicians. If outpatient rates are equal in the two communities, the higher hospitalization rate may be due to differences in physician practice styles.

Alternatively, Sadcom may have more severe injuries presenting to the emergency room, even though the rate of outpatient visits may not be higher than Onestate's. Severity of injury would, therefore, also need to be assessed.

6. Specific injury types may be increased: Examine rates of hospitalization by injury type (pedestrian injuries, drownings, poisonings, etc.) for the two populations.

7. Psycho-social factors: Obtain data on rates of alcoholism, foster care placement, violent crime, etc. for the two communities.

EXERCISE 2: EMERGENCY MEDICAL SERVICES

Interpreting Hospital-Based Data

To determine if emergency medical services were improving the outcome of spinal cord injury patients, a survey was undertaken. The medical directors of Spinal Cord Injury Centers (SCICs) in the United States were asked, What proportion of victims were arriving at their centers with severe injuries? The data from the SCICs were as follows:

	1984	*1994*
Severely injured (%)	70	40
Moderately injured (%)	30	60

The physicians believe that this 'substantial improvement' is primarily due to better care at the injury scene as a result of better trained attendants properly immobilizing patients and therefore preventing more severe injury.

Are there other explanations, besides better care at the scene, that could account for the above statistics?

ANSWERS

One possibility is that the proportion of people who suffer severe spinal cord injuries was reduced in the ten-year period. Since many spinal injuries are from motor vehicles, a reduction in the legal speed limit on highways, for example, would be expected to reduce severe spinal cord trauma.

Another possible explanation is that there has been a shifting of less-severely injured patients from local hospitals to SCICs. To illustrate, let us assume that 20 per cent of spinal cord injury patients have severe injuries (e.g. total paralysis) in both 1984 and 1994. Assume also that 10,000 people suffer spinal injuries in each year. By merely increasing the proportion of patients brought to SCICs rather than local hospitals, the distribution of mildly- and severely-injured can be altered:

1984

Condition of patients	Number (%) at scene	% transported to SCICs	Condition of patients at SCICs (%)
Severely injured	2,000 (20)	35	700 (69)
Moderately injured	8,000 (80)	4	320 (31)

1994

Condition of patients	Number (%) at scene	% transported to SCICs	Condition of patients at SCICs (%)
Severely injured	2,000 (20)	50	1,000 (40)
Moderately injured	8,000 (80)	19	1,500 (60)

In the above example, the quality of care at the scene remains exactly the same in 1984 and 1994. Yet the SCICs see a higher proportion of less-severely injured patients because the emergency transport patterns have changed.

EXERCISE 3: SOURCES OF DATA

The National Highway Traffic Safety Administration (NHTSA) wants to identify different ways to measure the impact of safety belt laws. They plan to award a one-year grant to review potential data sources and evaluate the usefulness of the data. The data can be local, state or national. Ideally, the data should be:
- available before and since enactment of a law requiring car occupants to wear seat belts;
- logically related to the consequences of crashes and seat belt use.

Obviously, you would use death-certificate data from each state to analyze whether motor vehicle death rates had fallen in specific age groups covered by seat belts laws. What other types of data could you examine?

ANSWERS

Among the 'candidate indicators' suggested by the NHTSA itself were the following:

A. Hospital- or Medical-related Data

1. Hospital emergency room records.
2. Hospital admission (or discharge) records.
3. Incidence or frequencies of head, brain, neck, spinal cord injuries; epilepsy, facial lacerations, fractures, or dental repairs.

4. Hospital bed-days or average hospital stay for motor-vehicle injuries.
5. Treatment costs: emergency room, hospital admissions, or rehabilitation.

B. Disability Data

1. Membership charges in organizations serving people disabled by crash injuries.
2. Sales volume of prostheses (artificial limbs) and adaptive devices for vehicles of disabled persons.
3. Reductions in organ donations of crash fatalities.

C. Police- or Emergency Medical Services-related Data

1. Collision and injury reports filed by police and drivers.
2. Ambulance records.

D. Employer Data

1. Lost man-days of work due to vehicle injuries.
2. Self-reports of belt use on health risk appraisals.

Insurance companies are another source of data: workmen's compensation claims for motor vehicle injuries, payments for medical services, disability payments, etc. Probably your list of potential data sources is even more extensive.

EXERCISE 4: INTERPRETING NATIONAL DATA*

Sri Lanka, formerly Ceylon, is an island republic, south of the Indian subcontinent. It has a population of 15.3 million (1983 estimate) and

---

* This exercise was adapted from material contained in: Berger, L. R. 1988. Suicides and pesticides in Sri Lanka. *American Journal of Public Health* **78**: 826–8.

covers 25,332 square miles. Rice is the main domestic crop. Major exports are tea, coconuts, rubber, textiles, petroleum products, and gems. The country's official language is Sinhala, Tamil and English are also spoken. The 1983 per capita GNP was $301. According to the 1981 Population Census, the literacy rate was 91 per cent for males and 82 per cent for females.

The most recent year for which computerized death certificate data was available was 1981. The information on causes of injury is recorded by ICDA E-codes ('E' standing for 'external causes of injury'). According to the Judicial Medical Officer of Sri Lanka's Department of Health (personal communication), death certificates are completed for an estimated 95 per cent of deaths. Some infant deaths in isolated areas of the country are the primary source of unreported deaths.

Hospital discharge data is collected by the Office of the Medical Statistician. Department of Census and Statistics, Ministry of Home Affairs. Only government hospitals (which account for approximately thirty per cent of hospital admissions) report this information. Private and military hospitals do not. Only the nature of injury (fracture, burn, contusion, etc.) is listed. E-coding is not performed.

Tables D.1, D.2, D.3 summarize the mortality data for males and females in Sri Lanka in 1981. Table 4, provides information on hospitalizations.

QUESTIONS

1. How important are injuries in Sri Lanka as compared to other health problems as a cause of death and as a reason for hospitalization?
2. What age- and sex- groups are at high risk of injuries?
3. What types of injury are most important as causes, of death at different ages?
4. With the information that there are 1,567,000 males and 1,547,000 females ages 15–24 years in Sri Lanka, calculate the death rate for suicides in this age group.
5. What data suggests the most likely method used to commit suicide in Sri Lanka?
6. Why this country have such an apparently high rate of suicide?

ANSWERS

1. Injuries account for 8.5 per cent of all female deaths and 14 per cent of all male deaths. There were nearly 2.5 million admissions to government hospitals with over 30,000 in-hospital deaths in 1984 (Table D.4). Injuries were 11.8 per cent of the admissions and 18.6 per cent of the in-hospital deaths.

2. In the 15 to 24 year old age group, the percentages of deaths that are injury-related are 53 per cent for females and 64 per cent for males.

3. Most remarkable is the proportion of injury-related deaths that are *suicides*: 47 per cent (1,509/3,199) for females of all ages and 41 per cent (2,892/7,096) for males (73 per cent and 59 per cent, respectively, for 15 to 24 year olds). Other categories of injury associated with large numbers of deaths are transportation (76 per cent of which are motor vehicle related), drownings, homicides and other violence, falls, and burns.

4. Both males and females have very high rates of suicide in Sri Lanka: the suicide rates by sex for ages 15–24 years are 74.9 per 100,000 for males and 60.9 for females. (Comparable rates in the United States are 20.2 and 4.3, respectively.)

5. *Pesticide poisonings* accounted for 42 per cent of all in-hospital, injury-related deaths for which a specific 'nature of injury' diagnosis was recorded.

6. That Sri Lanka's high suicide rate is merely an *artifact of over-reporting* is unlikely. Despite its economic difficulties, Sri Lanka has an excellent health services system and reporting of death is mandatory. The country's strong religious traditions would lead one to predict that suicides would be under- rather than over-reported.

The widespread *availability of liquid pesticides* in Sri Lanka makes them an attractive vehicle for suicide attempts. Approximately 700,000 kilograms of pesticides (including malathion in more than 200 formulations) are imported annually. Almost every rural grocery store has shelves full of many brands of pesticides in bottles of various sizes. Over 100 chemicals (including malathion in more than 120 formulations) are sold. Three-fourths of pesticide deaths in Sri Lanka are suicides.

Liquid preparations of pesticides can be lethal in minute doses.

The acute oral LD-50 for a 50-kilogram person ingesting certain pesticides in formulations recommended in Sri Lanka is less than *one ounce*. Organophosphorus compounds (parathion, malathion) are involved in a majority of poisonings. Mixtures of organophosphorus and organochlorine compounds are the most lethal: the in-hospital case-fatality rate for these ingestions in Sri Lanka is 33 per cent.

There are many psycho-social and economic factors that might contribute to suicide in Sri Lanka: the prolonged and violent civil strife between Sinhalese and Tamils, the clash of Western and traditional values, the recession which has struck agricultural economies particularly hard. Many of these factors will be extraordinarily difficult to alter in the immediate future. However, there is good reason to believe that restricting the availability of the lethal agent (pesticides) is likely to reduce the overall rate of suicide. When carbon monoxide was eliminated from coal gas in Birmingham, England, substitution of other forms of self-destruction occurred to some extent, but the overall suicide rate fell more than 50 per cent:

Many, if not the majority, of homicides and suicides are impulsive acts that will not be repeated. It is the lethality of the means at hand more than the planned intent of the persons involved that results in death.[9]

In 1983, a Registrar of Pesticides was appointed with authority to set regulations and standards for pesticides in Sri Lanka. There are many complicated issues to consider: What pesticides are currently used for control of insects, fungi, weeds, rodents, and parasites? Can less toxic chemicals be substituted for existing ones? What are the economic implications (for the country and for individual farmers) of limiting the availability of certain pesticides? The public health implications are also of great importance. However, perhaps the above data will encourage restrictions on the importation and sale of the most lethal pesticides.

REFERENCES

1. Manciaux, M., Romer, C. J. 1986. Accidents in children, adolescents and young adults: A major public health problem. *World Health Statistics Quarterly* **39**: 227–31.
2. The epidemiology of accident traumas and resulting disabilities. EURO Reports and Studies 57. Copenhagen: Regional Office for Europe, World Health Organization, 1982.

3. Principles for injury prevention in developing countries. Geneva: World Health Organization, 1985.
4. Abeyasekara, G. 1984. Sri Lanka's economy in 1984. *Economic Review* **10**: 4–14.
5. Annual Health Bulletin, Sri Lanka, 1983. Sri Lanka: Ministry of Health, 1984.
6. Youth Suicide in the United States, 1970–1980. Atlanta: Centers for Disease Control, Division of Injury Epidemiology and Control, 1986, p. 9.
7. Herath, H. M. S. S. D., Rajendra, M., Profile of accidents and episodes involving toxic chemicals in Sri Lanka. Background document, Intercountry Workshop on Chemical Safety, South East Asia Regional Office, WHO, New Delhi: 29 October–2 November 1984.
8. Gerard, B. M., Practical measures to reduce poisoning by agricultural pesticides in Sri Lanka. FAO/UNDP Project SRL/78/006, January 1983.
9. Robertson, L. S. 1983. Injuries: Causes, Control Strategies, and Public Policy. Lexington: Lexington Books.

Table D.1

Mortality Rates for the Five Leading Causes of Death by Age Group[*]
Sri Lanka, 1971–82

Cause of Death	Age Group (in Years)												
	<1	1–4	5–9	10–14	15–19	20–4	25–9	30–9	40–9	50–9	60–9	>70
Circulatory Diseases	–	–	–	6.9	10.8	17.7	25.3	46.4	118.3	289.0	598.3	1,109.0
Infectious Diseases	502.5	132.0	51.5	23.9	17.2	23.0	29.0	40.8	71.0	120.2	214.7	475.3
Respiratory Diseases	580.5	109.2	23.5	10.0	10.2	14.0	17.2	22.5	–	92.9	203.1	466.8
External Injury	–	–	22.8	34.0	74.5	101.0	88.2	73.8	77.0	90.5	–	–
CNS Diseases	–	29.3	–	8.9	10.2	–	–	–	–	–	252.4	946.6
Infant Perinatal Disorders	1,793.2	–	–	–	–	–	–	–	–	–	–	–
Malignancies	–	–	–	–	–	–	–	–	61.3	125.3	–	–
Nutritiolnal Deficiencies	152.3	69.9	17.3	–	–	–	–	–	–	–	–	–
Ill-defined Conditions	967.5	110.3	30.8	14.6	13.1	14.2	20.6	26.7	52.6	129.0	543.9	5,972.9
Total	4,513.3	521.7	185.6	114.6	157.2	221.7	245.3	306.8	552.8	1,120.6	2,554.4	6,358.9

[*] per 100,000 population.
Source: Sri Lanka Department of Census and Statistics.

Table D.2
External Causes of Death Registered in Sri Lanka, 1981 (Females)

	All Ages	<1	1-4	5-14	15-24	25-44	45-64	65-74	75
Transport	253	3	1	21	38	71	50	31	29
Accidental Poisoning	100	3	6	9	38	27	11	4	2
Falls	74	5	6	4	10	15	15	9	10
Fires/Flames	198	13	13	20	49	48	22	11	22
Natural and Environmental	76	2	4	18	21	19	7	3	2
Snakes/Lizards	182	3	14	47	42	41	28	5	2
Drowning	336	5	68	74	72	59	26	15	17
Other Accidents	132	24	4	17	16	26	23	7	5
Suicide	1,509	–	–	53	942	361	106	27	20
Homicide and Other Violence	339	25	14	20	69	131	46	22	12
Injuries (Total)	3,199	83	139	283	1,297	798	334	134	121
All Causes (Total)	37,663	5,632	1,994	1,230	2,444	3,757	6,139	5,722	10,738

Source: Registrar General's Office, Colombo.

Table D.3
External Causes of Death Registered in Sri Lanka, 1981 (Males)

	All Ages	<1	1-4	5-14	15-24	25-44	45-64	65-74	75
Transport	822	2	13	28	167	327	154	85	46
Accidental Poisoning	265	8	7	26	65	94	42	14	9
Falls	465	1	11	41	70	113	146	55	28
Fires/Flames	99	10	14	5	16	17	10	10	17
Natural & Environmental	159	5	12	20	35	38	33	5	11
Snakes/Lizards	329	4	20	64	72	92	53	16	8
Drowning	610	10	81	100	113	143	89	34	40
Other Accidents	426	23	25	28	84	129	84	32	21
Suicide	2,892	–	–	73	1,174	935	463	139	108
Homicide and Other Violence	1,029	21	23	28	206	422	232	61	35
Injuries (Total)	7,096	84	206	413	2,002	2,310	1,306	451	323
All Causes (Total)	50,818	6,875	1,933	1,507	3,109	5,731	10,995	8,386	12,273

Source: Registrar General's Office, Colombo.

Table D.4
Admissions to Government Hospitals for Injuries, Sri Lanka, 1984

Type of Injury	No. of Admissions	No. of In-hospital Deaths
Fractures	21,729	164
Dislocations, Sprains	10,616	5
Intracranial	7,730	458
Other Internal	2,232	130
Open Wounds	109,525	123
Dog Bites	4,861	5
Foreign Bodies	4,870	23
Burns	9,903	245
Poisonings Medicines	2,125	94
Pesticides	16,085	1,459
Other	7,032	697
Snake Bites	2,543	91
Total Injuries with Nature of Injury Recorded	199,251	3,494
Injuries with No Specific Diagnosis	93,369	2,136
Total Injuries	292,620	5,630
Total All Diagnoses	2,486,476	30,330

Source: Ministry of Health, Colombo.

EXERCISE 5: FALLS FROM TREES

Injury Prevention Strategies[*]

In the Cameroon, falls from palm trees are a common and serious problem. Teenagers and young adults climb the trees to harvest palm

---

[*] This exercise was adapted from an unpublished paper by Wansi Emmanuel, prepared during a course in Injury Epidemiology with Dr Dorothy Clemmer, Tulane School of Public Health.

nuts for oil production. The oil is widely used for cooking and is exported for industrial uses. Poultry feed is just one of the useful by-products from the palm nuts. Another palm-related industry is wine production. The wine tapper first climbs the trees to set a collection container. He later returns to retrieve the palm liquid.

Climbing is done with bare feet. Once at the top of the tree, the climber leans against a rope which passes around the tree and his waist. He carries under his shoulder a bag containing a machete (a long knife), often without a sheath. Each climber works alone.

Falls occur when the waist-strap breaks, when the worker stretches too far to pick a palm nut on a distant branch, when a branch breaks unexpectedly while the worker is holding it for support, and when the worker slips while climbing up or down the tree.

Using Dr Haddon's matrix and 10 technologic strategies (Chapter Six) as guide, what interventions can you suggest to reduce injuries from among the palm-tree workers?

ANSWERS

Some possible strategies for reducing the fall injuries are listed below. Obviously, some interventions will be more feasible than others: consider the barriers to introducing each of the proposed strategies.

- Launch an education campaign to make farmers more aware of fall hazards, simple safety measures, and first aid.
- Encourage climbers to work in groups, to look for hazards, provide emergency aid, remind each other of safety procedures, and increase productivity at the same time.
- Design and make available at miminal cost:
  a. work clothes equipped with a sturdy safety strap.
  b. shoes for climbing that will increase the grip on the trees.
  c. a scabbard (sheath) for the machete.
  d. a simple tool, perhaps a stick-blade-basket instrument for plucking palm nuts at a distance.
- Mechanize the work with a vehicle to lift people to the tops of trees.
- Introduce low-growing palm trees and provide incentives for planting them.
- Grow crops other than palms.

EXERCISE 6: HOW TO CRITIQUE AN INJURY RESEARCH ARTICLE

No person can possibly read all the articles that are published each year in any field. Unless you are reading a journal for leisure, choosing which articles to read should be based on their importance to you. However, an article worth reading does not necessarily reflect a high quality of research. It is therefore important to read articles actively and critically.

A useful approach to the literature is outlined in Table D.6. A valuable habit is to first ask yourself questions 1 and 2. What is the study about and why is it important? Then set the article aside and write down your thoughts in answer to the following question. If you were to conduct a study to answer the hypothesis or question posed in the article, and you had unlimited resources available, how would your study be structured? The ideal study is usually a randomized, controlled trial with strict criteria for enrollment and outcomes. After you have written down the elements of your hypothetical study, compare them to what is contained in the published article by answering the remaining questions in Table D.5.

Table D.5
An Outline to Critique a Research Article

1. What question or hypothesis does the study seek to answer?
2. Why is the question or hypothesis important?
3. What was actually done?
4. What was the experimental design: prospective? Randomized control group? Double blind?
5. Were the important terms unambiguously defined?
   a. case
   b. intervention
   c. outcomes
6. How comparable was the comparison group?
7. What are the results?
8. Are the authors' conclusions justified by the results?
9. Were the statistical methods stated? Was sample size discussed?
10. What questions did the study raise that further research might address?
11. How is the study relevant to preventing injuries?

To practice this approach, read the following paragraphs as if they were a summary of a study that had actually been published. Then answer the questions below.

Car Safety Seat Study

The use of car safety seats is vital for the safe transportation of infants and young children in automobiles. In the general population, only 5 per cent of infants are transported in car safety seats. To determine if pediatricians can increases car seat use for infants, the following study was performed.

The study population consisted of 100 pregnant women referred by their obstetricians for a prenatal visit by a pediatrician at Caremore Hospital. Each woman spent 30 minutes with the pediatrician, discussing topics such as circumcision, breast feeding, and plans for delivery. Also, each woman was told about the importance of car safety seats for their infants.

Three months after delivery, the pediatrician contacted each mother by telephone. All 100 women were contacted and asked:

EXERCISE 7: INFANT CAR SEAT STUDY

(1) Did you purchase a car safety seats for your baby?
(2) Do you use the car seat regularly and appropriately?

Twenty-five per cent of the women answered 'Yes' to both questions. This five-fold increase (5 per cent vs 25 per cent) should prompt pediatricians to incorporate education about car safety seats into their regular discussions with new parents.

QUESTIONS

1. What is the hypothesis of this study?
2. If you were to design an 'ideal' study to test the hypothesis, how would you do it?
3. How do the methods in your ideal study compare with the above study?

4. Do you agree with the conclusions of the above study?

ANSWERS

1. HYPOTHESIS: Prenatal interviews by pediatricians can increase the proportion of infants appropriately transported in car safety seats.
2. Elements of an 'ideal' study:
   a. Pregnant women would be randomized to intervention and control groups.
   b. A standardized intervention would be provided: a structured interview and printed handouts.
   c. The outcome of the study would be direct observations of car seat use, as when the parents brought their infants to the pediatrician's office for a regular well-child visit.
   d. Criteria for 'appropriate use' of the car seats would be specified at the outset: the car seat would have to be strapped to the automobile seat with seat belts; the infants would have to be harnessed to the car seat.
3. In the 'reported' study:
   a. A comparison is made with restraint use in the general population (5 per cent). There are no controls from the same population that is seen in the obstetrical practices. The latter are likely to be more highly educated and wealthier than the general population, and therefore more likely to purchase car safety seats with or without prenatal advice.
   b. The intervention was not standardized. Different pediatricians might have provided different advice and information.
   c. The outcome of the study relied on mothers reporting by telephone whether or not they purchased car safety seats and 'used them regularly and appropriately'. The terms 'regularly' and 'appropriately' were not defined. Also, reported use or compliance is often very unreliable, since individuals know what the interviewer (in this case, their family's own pediatrician) wants to hear.
4. The decision about whether to discuss car safety in paediatri-

cians' offices cannot be based on the poorly-constructed study described above. Since motor vehicle crashes are the leading cause of death in childhood in HICs, car seats are readily available to nearly all families, and counseling about car seats is not very time-consuming; most pediatricians in the United States discuss car safety as part of routine preventive care.

FURTHER READINGS

1. Sackett, D. L. 1981. How to read clinical journals: I. Why to read them and how to start reading them critically. *Canadian Medical Association Journal* **124**: 555–8.
2. Sackett, D. L. 1981. How to read clinical journals: V. To distinguish useful from useless or even harmful therapy. *Canadian Medical Association Journal* **124**: 1156–61.
3. Sackett, D. L., Haynes, R. B., Tugwell, P. 1985. Clinical Epidemiology: A Basic Science for Clinical Medicine. Little-Brown, Boston.
4. Riegelman, R. K. 1981. Studying a Study and Testing a Test: How to read the medical literature. Little-Brown, Boston.
5. Berger, L. R., Saunders, S., Armitage, K. et al. 1984. Promoting the use of car safety devices for infants: An intensive health education approach. *Pediatrics* **74**: 16–19.

EXERCISE 8:   PREPARING AN INJURY RESEARCH PROPOSAL IN EPIDEMIOLOGY

Many readers will submit research proposals to their own academic institutions or to funding agencies. In this exercise, participants are asked to prepare an epidemiology research proposal on an injury topic of their choice.

This exercise may be done in a group during a half-day workshop or as an individual assignment over the course of a semester. Depending on the background of the participants, and on the time provided for completion of the exercise, some or all of the items in Table D.6 can be addressed. All proposals should at a minimum address items A through D: Topic, Importance, Background, and Methods.

Table D.6
Outline for an Injury Research Proposal

A. Topic:

What major questions or hypotheses does the study seek to address?

B. Importance:

Why is the topic important? How will the research results be applied
to reducing injuries? What groups will be interested in the findings?

C. Background:

What information is already available about the injury problem in the
target community: its extent, severity, and high-risk groups?
What articles have been published about prevalence, causes, and
possible countermeasures?

D. Methods:

What type of study do you propose?
descriptive, hypothesis-testing, community trial
case-control, cohort, cross-sectional
prospective or retrospective
What kind of data will you collect?

Interviews	Clinical examinations
Laboratory tests	Direct observations
Review of existing records	

What are the 'criteria for inclusion'?
How is an 'injury' defined? Are occupational, motor vehicle,
domestic, and intentional injuries (rape, suicide, homicide, assaults,
child abuse) included?
What range of injury severity (deaths, hospitalizations, out-patient
visits) will be covered?
What ages will be included?
How and by whom will the data be collected?
What sampling procedures will be used (how the target population will
be selected, number of subjects, representativeness of the sample)?
What comparison data (e.g., census, general hospital admissions)
will be used?
What denominators will be used for calculating rates?
How will the data be analyzed? Provide examples of calculations, tables.

Why is the proposed method of research an appropriate one? What are its possible limitations and how will they be addressed?

E. Personnel:

Describe the project staff including their roles, qualifications, and the percentage of time each will devote to the project.

F. Human Studies:

If human subjects are involved, describe how the study will ensure confidentiality and protect against physical, psychological, or social risks.

G. Timetable:

Consider the planning phase, training interviewers and staff, conducting a pilot survey, data collection and analysis, and writing the final report.

H. Budget:

Estimate costs of personnel, equipment, travel, communication, etc.

EXERCISE 9: AN OUTBREAK OF DYSURIA AMONG INDUSTRIAL WORKERS*

On 28 March 1978, a local board of health in a small town received a telephone call from an emergency-room physician in a nearby community hospital. The physician reported that 11 workers from the same polyurethane foam factory had come as a group to the emergency room at 9 a.m. that Monday morning. All the workers complained of trouble urinating, although each of them produced a normal urine specimen.

QUESTIONS

1. If you were on the staff of the local health department, what would you do to pursue this report?

---

* This exercise is adapted from a case study by Dr Kathleen Kreiss contained in: *A Joint Publication on Teaching Epidemiology in Occupational Health*: NIOSH/WHO, May, 1987. It is based on published material in *Reference 1*. Used with permission.

The eight men and three women, who had sought medical attention, had suffered for several months from difficulty in starting their urine stream, which was weak and difficult to maintain. The plant manager confirmed that many more employees had similar problems and that two employees had had surgery for inability to urinate. He wanted to cooperate in every way since his earlier efforts to have the bathrooms cleaned and inspected had not solved the problem being experienced by employees.

The factory manufactured polyurethane foam seats for automobiles. The plant had two parallel production lines, as well as finishing, supply, storage, laboratory, and clerical areas. At the head of each production line, the ingredients of the foam were compounded: toluene di-isocyanate, polyols, fire retardants, and a catalyst. This mixture was poured into open waxed molds, and a cover was placed on top of the mold as the foam expanded. The closed mold was then passed through an oven, after which the cured foam cushion was removed and conveyed to the adjacent finishing room. There, the foam was trimmed, inspected, and bagged in polyethylene for shipping. The mold and its cover were stripped of excess foam, sprayed with wax, and fitted with nets and wires for the structural support of the next cushion.

The major building block of polyurethane is toluene di-isocyanate (TDI), which causes occupational asthma in a small percentage of workers who become sensitized, and which may cause excessive decrements in lung function in non-sensitized workers, comparable in magnitude to the yearly decrement caused by cigarette smoking.[2] Neither TDI nor other chemicals used in the plant were known to cause urinary symptoms. However, since a large number of employees seemed to have similar urinary complaints, further investigation was warranted.

2.   How would you investigate this apparent outbreak?

The only new chemical which had been introduced in the preceding year was a catalyst, dimethylaminopropenenitrile (DMAPN). The catalyst was introduced on one production line in August 1977 and was used irregularly until December of that year. From December 1977, both assembly lines had used the catalyst. Since DMAPN was a leading suspect for a chemical culprit, the management removed it from production on 29 March 1978.

An epidemiological survey was started a week later. All available employees completed a questionnaire and gave a urine and a blood sample. A case of bladder dysfunction was defined as an employee who had experienced any two of the following four symptoms: hesitancy, straining to void, decreased force of the stream, or increased duration of urination.

3. a) Why was a case definition made?
   b) Who could serve as controls?

Of the 208 employees, 104 met the case definition. The attack rate among the 166 persons exposed to DMAPN in the production or finishing areas was 63 per cent. No cases occurred among the remaining 42 employees. There were 20 cases (55.6 per cent) among 36 exposed women and 84 cases (65.5 per cent) among 130 exposed men.

Many different symptoms were reported (Table D.7). Patients complained of having to press on the lower abdomen to begin urination. Several persons said they completely lost the urge to urinate. Others described increased frequency of urination, particularly as their conditions improved. Some lost urethral sensation or had urethral burning. Most had vague abdominal discomfort that they did not associate with bladder distension. Sexual difficulties occurred in 23 persons classed as cases and six non-cases. Thirteen 'cases had upper extremity numbness.

4. a) What might be the mechanism of this set of complaints? How would you confirm your hypothesis?
   b) What is the design of this study, case-control, cohort, or other?

The epidemic curve is shown in Figure D.1.

5. Does the epidemic curve support the suspicion that DMAPN caused the outbreak of bladder dysfunction? What other information would be helpful?

6 Having concluded the epidemiological survey, what would you do next?

ANSWERS

1. The information given is not sufficient to make a medical diagnosis or to relate the workers, complaints to a workplace exposure. To verify the complaints, the available medical and demographic information must be collected. This is most easily accomplished by reviewing the medical records of the workers

Table D.7
Urinary Complaints

Symptoms	Cases	Controls
Increased duration	102/104	1/104
Hesitancy	98/104	0/104
Need to strain	98/104	0/104
Decreased stream	94/104	4/104
Subjective retention	70/102	4/104
Dysuria	70/104	13/104
Abdominal discomfort	61/103	6/104
Urgency	47/104	3/104
Decreased frequency	47/104	23/104
Increased frequency	44/104	23/104
Urethral discharge	19/104	2/80
Nocturia	15/104	10/104
Gross haematuria	12/104	4/104

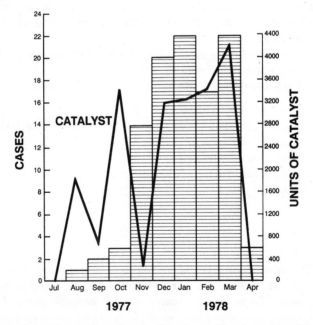

Figure D.1: The number of cases of workers with urinary complaints
rose and fell with the amount of catalyst used at the factory.

who were seen in the emergency room. These records contain age, sex, complaints, results of physical examination and laboratory evaluation of urine and other biological specimens, and identity of patients, should further information be required. In addition, some information might be available about whether the complaints stemmed from an acute process, with 11 employees being affected simultaneously and coming as a group from work, or alternatively, from a chronic condition, in which case the implications of 11 persons meeting as a group at the emergency room after a weekend's respite are different. In fact, the latter was the case, and many more employees than 11 had agreed to meet at the hospital. They wanted to dramatize the work-related character of their complaints, which had been ignored by private physicians whom they had consulted individually.

In addition to ascertaining more about the medical aspect of the worker's complaints, information must be sought about the work environment of the polyurethane foam plant. This information can be sought from the patients and from the management. The factory management may be able to confirm whether there is an epidemic in the workplace based on absenteeism or complaints to a medical department (if any). The management is usually the only source of a list of workplace chemicals and a detailed account of changes in production process, ventilation, and industrial hygiene measurements of workplace exposures.

2. Three simple means of investigation exist for characterizing an outbreak of a new occupational disease: an epidemiological survey, referral of severely affected persons to medical specialists for detailed diagnostic testing, and correlation of changes in production processes or measurements of chemical exposure with the occurrence of illness.

The goals of an epidemiological survey are to establish who is affected, where in the production process, and when. Characterizing who is affected requires questions concerning age, sex, job category, personal hygiene, shift worked, duration of employment, absenteeism, and presence of specific symptoms. A case definition must be formulated for the purpose of comparing affected employees (cases) with unaffected employees (controls) for attributes or risk factors for illness. Locating onset of complaints in time may also give a valuable clue to which changes in production processes may be responsible. Latency of the illness after first exposure to the plant might be determined by analysis of the symptom experience of recently hired employees.

Appropriate diagnostic testing, in conjunction with a questionnaire survey or by referral to medical specialists, requires hypothesis about the nature of the disorder. In this outbreak, the investigators were puzzled because the emergency-room physician had made no diagnosis and the available data were not compatible with infection or prostatic obstruction especially considering that some of those affected were women.

No known industrial chemical produced urinary retention on a pharmacological basis and persons complained of symptoms persisting over a week-long plant closure during a blizzard. No known neurotoxin affected the bladder preferentially. It appeared that detailed testing by neurologists and urologists was the most promising line. Another group of investigators chose to do intravenous pyelograms as well as to evaluate the disorder.[3] Of course, hypothesis about the nature of the illness must be formulated before the design of the symptom portion of the questionnaire.

Production records are useful in several ways: they can indicate any new chemicals which may have been introduced in the preceding year and where and in what amount they had been used. Also, exposure to chemicals, and resulting incidence rates, can vary by shift and by assembly line.

3. a) In this setting the assessment of disease status must be based on a variety of symptoms, which should be condensed into a single summary variable as to whether each individual was ill or well. A case definition, which is to a large extent arbitrary, is one method for doing this. This approach allows us to divide the population into cases and non-cases, or controls, in order to look for differences in characteristics which may be valuable clues as to risk factors or protective factors for disease. Had our investigation measured some quantitative measure of dysfunction, we might have chosen to retain the continuous data in our analysis.

   b) Non-cases can serve as controls. Another approach is to divide the population into an 'at-risk' group and an 'unexposed' group.

The at-risk group includes all employees who worked in the production or finishing areas, who were assumed to be exposed to DMAPN. These at-risk employees are then compared with employees working in non-manufacturing areas such as the warehouse. This means of analysis is that of a cohort study, rather than a case-control study. Both means of analysis use a comparison group, or control group. In a cohort study, the exposed group is compared to the unexposed group for disease outcome. In a case-control study, the case group is compared to the non-case group for risk factors.

4. a) Occupational neuropathies which affect the peripheral nerves usually cause numbness or tingling (sensory changes) or weakness (motor changes) in the hands or feet. The bladder nerves are part of the peripheral nervous system, but are autonomic rather than somatic. Some toxic neuropathies have autonomic effects. For example, acrylamide causes abnormal sweating. Although only a small number of persons (13/104) complained of extremity numbness, suggesting a peripheral neuropathy, the mechanism of the urinary and sexual dysfunction was undoubtedly neurological. A sensory neuropathy was suggested by abnormal urethral sensation and loss of the sense of bladder fullness. A motor neuropathy was suggested by the difficulty in initiating and maintaining the urine stream.

    Eight symptomatic employees were referred for neurologic testing two and a half weeks after DMAPN was removed from production. Seven of them had neurological abnormalities of the distal lower extremities on physical examination. Nerve conduction tests on peroneal and sural (lower leg) nerves and on pudendal nerves showed at least one abnormal measurement in four of the eight. Five patients lacked the detrusor reflex which empties the bladder in a coordinated fashion. Two additional patients had a high sensory threshold for bladder filling. These findings on neurological testing and cystometrograms are consistent with a neuropathy affecting the bladder nerves.

    b) In this study, prevalence information was collected from 208 of 213 current workers. Five workers refused to participate. Because the information on exposure and disease was collected simultaneously, this study is cross-sectional. Only by chance do the number of cases (104) equal the number of non-cases.

5. A rough exposure-response relation is suggested by the amount

of catalyst used in monthly production and the incidence of new cases (Figure D.1). Exposure-response relationships are an important finding in support of causal association.

6. There are many appropriate next steps:

   a) Prevention of further cases of an occupational disease is the justification of all the investigative steps. When the cause of an outbreak of occupational disease is clear, control of the disease is usually clear. In this instance, the outbreak was terminated rapidly when the catalyst was removed from production. The producer voluntarily stopped selling the catalyst. In other instances, engineering controls and personnel protective equipment might be appropriate preventive measures, if substitution of chemical catalysts had not been possible. In that instance, animal toxicological studies might be needed to determine safe levels of exposure.

   b) A scientific and ethical responsibility is to see whether this epidemic was repeated elsewhere. The scientific responsibility illustrates another criterion for causality in epidemiological association: consistency of findings among investigators. This epidemic was a newly described association of a chemical exposure with a new kind of neuropathy. Another group of investigators had similar findings in a polyurethane foam plant in Maryland.[3] In the absence of a known similar outbreak, other users of the chemical can often be identified through the producer or with the assistance of governmental authorities (in the USA, the Occupational Safety and Health Administration or the National Institute for Occupational Safety and Health).

   c) Follow-up of persons classed as cases is important to determine the natural history of the disease and the efficacy of any treatment. In this outbreak, 51 per cent of the cases noted symptomatic improvement at the time of the survey (which was 8 to 13 days after removal of DMAPN from production). An additional 21 per cent of the cases said they were back to normal. Three months later, 76 per cent of the previous cases were asymptomatic, and the remainder reported improvement. However, some abnormalities were present at two-year follow-up in later groups.[4]

In the case of some industrial neurotoxins, treatment may be efficacious. For example, physicians try to accelerate the excretion of lead with disodiumedetale and of chlordecone (Kepone) with cholestyramine. The neurological effects of carbon monoxide poisoning are treated by the administration of oxygen. Unfortunately, for most occupational neuropathies caused by chemicals there is no known treatment.[5]

REFERENCES

1. Kreiss, K. et al. 1980. Neurological dysfunction of the bladder in workers exposed to dimethylaminopropenenitrile. *JAMA* **243**: 741–5.
2. Diem, J. E. et al. 1982. Five-year longitudinal study of workers employed in a new toluene di-isocyanate manufacturing plant. *American Review of Respiratory Disease* **126**: 420–8.
3. Keogh, J. P., Pestronk, A., Wertheimer, D., Moreland, R. 1980. An epidemic of urinary retention caused by dimethylaminopropenenitrite. *JAMA* **243**: 746–9.
4. Baker, E. L. et al. 1981. Follow-up studies of workers with bladder neuropathy caused by exposure to dimethylaminopropenenitrite. *Scandinavian Journal of Work, Environment and Health* **7**: suppl. 4, 54–9.
5. Spencer, P. S., Schaumburg, H. H. (eds). 1980. *Experimental and clinical neurotoxicology.* Baltimore, Williams and Wilkins.

Index